A Manual Therapist's Surface Anatomy and Palpation Skills

M000275308

I dedicate this book in loving memory of my mother Joan and my father David. I would also like to generously thank my understanding wife Annabel and our treasure Sophia for their patience and understanding as always

David Byfield

I dedicate this book to my wife Laurel with eternal gratitude for her commitment, love and support; and for having the opportunity to share in the joy of raising and nurturing our children, Melissa and Ted

Stuart Kinsinger

Commissioning editor: Heidi Allen
Development editor: Robert Edwards
Desk editor: Claire Hutchins
Production Controller: Chris Jarvis
Cover designer: Greg Harris

A Manual Therapist's Guide to Surface Anatomy and Palpation Skills

David Byfield BSc(Hons) DC MPhil FCC(Orth)
Welsh Institute of Chiropractic
University of Glamorgan
Pontypridd
Wales
UK

Stuart Kinsinger BSc DC FCCRS(c)
Canadian Memorial Chiropractic College
Toronto
Ontario
Canada

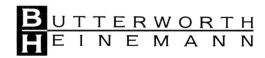

OXFORD   AUCKLAND   BOSTON   JOHANNESBURG   MELBOURNE   NEW DELHI

Butterworth-Heinemann
An imprint of Elsevier Science

© 2002, Elsevier Science Ltd. All rights reserved.

The right of David Byfield and Stuart Kinsinger to be identified as authors
of this work has been asserted by them in accordance with the Copyright,
Designs and Patents Act 1988

No part of this publication may be reproduced, stored in a retrieval system,
or transmitted in any form or by any means, electronic, mechanical, photocopying,
recording or otherwise, without either the prior permission of the publishers
(Permissions Manager, Elsevier Science Ltd, Robert Stevenson House,
1–3 Baxter's Place, Leith Walk, Edinburgh EH1 3AF), or a licence permitting
restricted copying in the United Kingdom issued by the Copyright Licensing Agency,
90 Tottenham Court Road, London W1T 4LP.

First published 2002

ISBN 0 7506 4484 2

British Library Cataloguing in Publication Data
A catalogue record for this book is available from the British Library

Library of Congress Cataloguing in Publication Data
A catalogue record for this book is available from the Library of Congress

Designed and typeset by Keyword Typesetting Services Ltd, Wallington, Surrey
Printed and bound in Great Britain by The Bath Press, Avon

The
Publisher's
policy is to use
**paper manufactured
from sustainable forests**

Contents

List of contributors   vii

Foreword   ix

Preface   xi

Acknowledgements   xiii

Introduction   xv
David Byfield and Stuart Kinsinger

1   Diagnostic palpation and anatomical
    landmark location – clinical concepts and
    the evidence   1
    David Byfield, Matthew Clancy and Vanessa Kelly

2   Basic postural observation skills   35
    David Byfield

3   Basic lumbopelvic palpation and landmark
    identification skills   45
    David Byfield

4   Basic thoracic spine palpation and landmark
    identification skills   73
    Stuart Kinsinger

5   Basic cervicothoracic and occiput palpation and
    landmark identification skills   79
    Stuart Kinsinger

6   Landmark location and palpation skills for the
    lower extremity   87
    David Byfield

7   Basic palpation and anatomical landmark
    identification skills for the upper
    extremity   133
    Stuart Kinsinger

Index   169

Contributors

David Byfield BSc(Hons), DC, MPhil, FCC(Orth)
Senior Lecturer
Welsh Institute of Chiropractic
University of Glamorgan
Pontypridd
Wales, UK

Stuart Kinsinger BSc, DC, FCCRS(c)
Assistant Professor
Chair, Department of Chiropractic Principles and
Practice
Canadian Memorial Chiropractic College
Toronto, Ontario
Canada

Matthew Clancy BSc(Hons), DC
Welsh Institute of Chiropractic
University of Glamorgan
Pontypridd
Wales, UK

Vanessa Kelly BSc(Hons), DC
Welsh Institute of Chiropractic
University of Glamorgan
Pontypridd
Wales, UK

Foreword

The acquisition of psychomotor skills is a complex activity taking many years to move from the novice to the experienced professional having achieved mastery of the subject. For the Doctor of Chiropractic and other practitioners of manual therapy, it is essential to demonstrate the knowledge, skills and attitude necessary to claim competence in practice. Although perhaps most closely identified with the care of the spine, Doctors of Chiropractic manage the health of their patients by utilizing a variety of investigative methods and therapeutic options applied where clinically indicated to the entire body.

The development of an individual's clinical decision-making ability is greatly supported by instructional methods designed to integrate knowledge and skills with their application delivered in the appropriate professional manner. Drs Byfield and Kinsinger have recognized this need through their years of experience in the provision of education for chiropractors. There is undoubtedly much value in information focused on specific anatomical regions and specific clinical needs. This text, however, provides a unique opportunity for the development of skills using a methodical approach underpinned by strong anatomical knowledge and applied globally with an understanding of the needs of the patient.

Readers will certainly be provided with a strong insight into the complexities associated with current education and training in psychomotor skills. They will appreciate the meticulous attention to detail demonstrated by these exceptional and experienced authors. This text will become essential reading for both the undergraduate and postgraduate healthcare professional dedicated to maintaining the highest standards of psychomotor skill acquisition and performance. Patients will be the beneficiaries of the most skilful approach to their care and wellbeing.

Dr Susan King DC DHSM MBS
Head, Welsh Institute of Chiropractic
at the University of Glamorgan,
Wales, United Kingdom

Preface

Educating undergraduate students requires patience and commitment. This is a slow and evolving process that provides future health practitioners with those essential competencies necessary to begin a life long career of caring for patient' needs. Professional education also establishes a solid foundation for continued learning and ongoing clinical experience; essential qualities for the life long learner. The basis of professional development is underpinned by core psychomotor palpatation and observational skills combined with a strong knowledge base and current scientific evidence rationale. Clinical observation, diagnostic palpation and manipulative therapeutics are intimately linked as the fundamental components of all manual therapeutic disciplines including, among many others, chiropractic, physical therapy, massage therapy and acupuncture. It is, therefore, crucial that undergraduate students understand the clinical importance of these principal skills including the time required assimilating the basic rudimentary skills of postural analysis, anatomical landmark location, joint play and end play examination.

This textbook provides a systematic and practical approach to presenting these essential observation and palpation skills to prepare the student for more advanced instruction concerning physical examination and manual therapeutics. The book methodically reviews the surface anatomy and provides an organized approach for locataing osseous and soft tissue landmarks relating to the major extremity joints (foot/ankle, knee, hip, shoulder girdle, elbow and wrist/hand) and all regions of the spine (cervical, thoracic, lumbar, pelvic).

The book also instructs key joint play and end play analysis procedures for all extremity and spinal joints. This provides a practical approach to palpation instruction and anatomical review as preparation for learning manipulative procedures for all regions of the spine and pelvis and extremity joints later during undergraduate training. Those ethical issues affecting the beginning student learning palpation skills are also dealt with.

There is no substitute for the fundamentals required in developing clinical practice skills particularly those required by a primary contact health practitioner. The entire basis of practice life and clinical success, to a great extent, revolves around the educational encounter experienced in the early undergraduate years. These may be painstaking at times and frustrating but a necessary process during professional development.

One of the primary reasons for writing this textbook was to fill a void in the instructional literature for teaching complex manual psychomotor skills used in the manual therapy disciplines. Though written by chiropractors that are actively engaged in teaching these skills to their students, many of the methods depicted in the text are common to a number of professional groups utilizing manual skills. The intent of the text is to present a simple yet effective instructional manual dedicated to basic anatomical and palpation concepts.

David Byfield
Welsh Institute of Chiropractic
University of Glamorgan

Stuart Kinsinger
Canadian Memorial Chiropractic College

Acknowledgements

We would like to thank Mike Davies, Media Services, University of Glamorgan Learning Resources and his staff including Chris Pascos and Cath Evans for their professionalism and patience during the photo shoot session and film processing. We would also like to acknowledge Lee Wickham, our model, for his participation in this project and wish him success in his chiropractic career. We would also like to recognize Dr Matt Clancy and Dr Vanessa Kelly for their contribution to the content and editing of Chapter 1. We would also like to endorse Atlas Clinical Ltd, UK for donating the chiropractic table and motion palpation station used during the photo session. A final thanks goes to Heidi Allen and Claire Hutchins for their patience and commitment to this project from the start.

Introduction

David Byfield and Stuart Kinsinger

Training for a career as a health care provider involves the understanding and learning of professionalism and professional conduct. A professional relationship is, by definition and practice, quite different from personal or casual relationships. The clinician is obligated and required to act and think carefully when involved with the patient/client. Standards of practice and clinical behaviours are regulated worldwide by all professional groups. Foremost in intent is the protection of the public, which the health care professional serves. Inappropriate behaviour by a health care provider towards the patient/client results in significant and severe penalties, in addition to the harm suffered by the client. In the initial process of learning palpation skills, it is essential that students understand and apply professional conduct at all times.

CLINICAL ISSUES

Palpation is the premier and most commonly employed examination technique used by all manual practitioners (Figure 1). More clinical information is obtained by palpation than any other method and it forms the foundation on which the others are considered. It takes a great deal of practice to develop proficiency at both the touching or contact aspect and the interpretation of what the 'touch' means. The skilled palpator is one who has learned the ability to discriminate tactually, focus mentally and integrate this combination of information. The most sensitive 'tools of the trade' for this purpose are the thumb pad and the finger pads of the first and second digits (Figure 2).

The student soon learns during the palpation of soft tissues the differences in skin texture and temperature, muscle tone and consistency, and tenderness to touch, when comparing various anatomical areas among different colleagues. Palpation of bony landmarks reveals contours and alignment, potential anomalies and tenderness to touch. Bony and joint palpation can be either performed as *static palpation*, or involve moving the anatomical part through a range of motion, termed *motion palpation* (*subdivided into joint play and end play and other assessory joint motions*). Moving

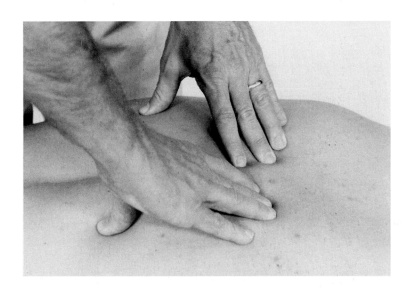

Fig. 1 Palpation examination

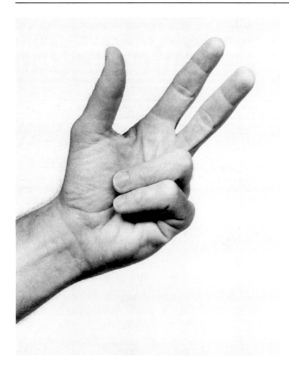

Fig. 2 Palpation 'tools of the trade'

the structure requires an even greater level of comprehension for not only feeling the tactile sensations, but also an appreciation for the quality and quantity of the motion.

The skilled palpator also has learned what is too much pressure and too little. Less touch is required when palpating those landmarks which are more superficial. The early learner tends to use either too much or too little pressure with too much pressure causing discomfort in his or her partner. Too little pressure does not allow the examiner to palpate the landmark properly and gives the partner little assurance of the palpator's competence. Sensitivity to your partner's comfort is a most critical component when learning palpation skills.

The skilled palpator must have an extremely good command of basic musculoskeletal anatomy. Full knowledge of the complexity of the skeletal system provides the early palpator with a good foundation to be able to learn the psychomotor skills as well as reasonably accurate landmark location. Being able to visualize and image mentally the structures under assessment may enhance the development of these important examination skills.

TOUCH ISSUES

For the newcomer learning the various aspects of professionalism, many concerns centre around the issue of touching the client. Touch is a way of showing compassion and a form of communication. These powerful qualities facilitate a closer connection in the therapist/client relationship when used in a careful, considerate way with the client's consent; but when used inappropriately, cause harm, in both physical and non-physical ways. This 'hands on' contact approach in a clinical context may in fact enhance recovery and provide positive patient outcomes.

Just as there are different kinds of touch, there are different perceptions of touch; some being appropriate and others perceived as inappropriate. The clinician must realize that good intentions are not sufficient, as the patient's family history and cultural milieu have shaped his or her perception of the reality of this touching event. As you, the student are being palpated, you will feel the different kinds of touch: firm, soft, hard, painful, gentle, soothing, careless, sensitive, assertive, dominating, tentative, assured, deliberate, clammy, poking, prodding, cold, warm, trembling, uncertain, disrespectful, respectful.

The violation of one's personal boundaries most often occurs through inappropriate touching. Because the intention of the therapist may be perceived as very different from the perception of your client, open communication between therapist and client is paramount. Routinely ask your partner for feedback on your palpation technique and report accurately and specifically both those positive and negative perceptions. Make this dialogue a regular part of the learning process as you learn palpation skills. These verbal skills and a keen awareness of these doctor–patient boundaries are extremely important aspects of professional training and development.

ETHICAL AND LEGAL ISSUES

No one has the right to be touched without consent first being given, even in a professional educational environment. While consent to participate may appear automatic in a professional educational institution, take care to be sensitive to your partner's feelings and concerns. These attitudes will be translated directly into your professional life and form the basis for codes and standards of practice as set down in statutory documentation. Realize that consent can and may also be withdrawn by the client. As a novice palpator, be aware of any assumptions held regarding this issue. In most jurisdictions any touch or other procedure performed without consent first being obtained is considered assault. This applies equally to the health care professional as to the lay person.

The professional has a duty to, without exception or reservation, consider the needs, health and well being of the client above the needs and desires of him- or herself.

Notwithstanding, professionals must suspend their own personal beliefs in the best interest of the patient at all times. This is one of the hallmark features of being a professional, with others including beneficence, non-malficience, respect, autonomy and justice.

INTERPERSONAL ISSUES

Practising good habits as a student learner assures a future successful professional practice. Since palpa-

tion is done with the fingers and hands, always wash up before and after the palpation skills class (Figure 3). Keep the fingernails and cuticles neat and clean. Remove any jewelry, which may interfere with your or your partner's learning experience. Good hygiene facilitates the learning of palpation skills due to your close physical proximity and the many hours needed to learn this most useful professional skill (Figure 4). Taking care in this area reaps many rewards both in student life and professional practice.

Professionals are held to a higher standard in ethics and behaviour. Learning palpatory skills is an excellent forum for understanding the concepts correlating these ethical behaviours as a student, and enjoying a successful career as a health care provider.

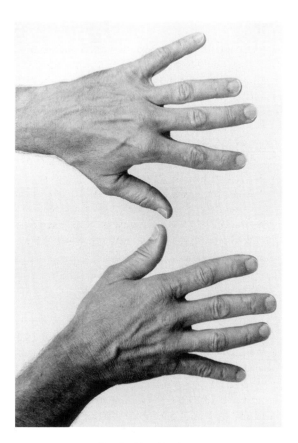

Fig. 3   Hand hygiene

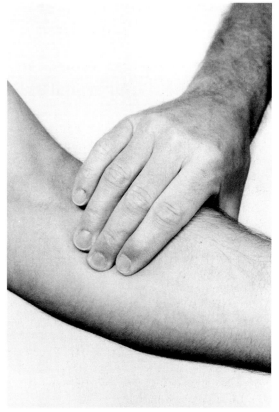

Fig. 4   Good hygiene facilitates learning process

Diagnostic palpation and anatomical landmark location – clinical concepts and the evidence

David Byfield, Matthew Clancy and Vanessa Kelly

INTRODUCTION

Palpation of the spine is arguably the most common investigative procedure used in the examination of the musculoskeletal system (Alley, 1983; Russell, 1983; Deboer et al., 1985; Harvey and Byfield, 1991; Panzer, 1992; Walker and Buchbinder, 1997; McKenzie and Taylor, 1997; French et al., 2000; O'Haire and Gibbons, 2000). Specifically, motion palpation is considered to be the most frequently employed diagnostic technique used by all practitioners of spinal manipulative therapy to identify both normal and abnormal spinal joint mobility parameters (Johnston, 1975; Breen, 1977; Russell, 1983; Jull et al., 1988; Mootz et al., 1989; Burton et al., 1990; Panzer, 1992). Furthermore, palpation techniques are considered an essential skill and an important procedure for identifying specific intervertebral segments targeted for manipulative intervention (Alley, 1983; Boline et al., 1988; Herzog et al., 1989; Hubka and Phelan, 1994; Haas et al., 1995a; Walker and Buchbinder, 1997). Moreover, the ability to distinguish accurately between normal and hypomobile spinal motion segments is a clinical asset, particularly when the therapy being administered has a mobility enhancing effect (Panzer, 1992). Nevertheless, despite the heavy reliance placed upon palpation findings, there is very little objective research evidence which establishes motion palpation as either a valid or reliable diagnostic method

and/or outcome measure (Keating, 1989a; Haas, 1991a). Most, if not all, investigations to date have failed to demonstrate acceptable inter-examiner reproducibility and confirmation of validity is scarce (Alley, 1983; Jansen and Nansel, 1988; Keating, 1989a; Haas, 1991a; Breen, 1992). Most reliability studies have been primarily concerned with relating palpation findings to the presence of spinal complaints and with intra- and inter-examiner agreement in both symptomatic and asymptomatic populations (Kaltenborn and Lindahl, 1969; Gonnella et al., 1982; Johnston, 1982; DeBoer et al., 1985; Potter and Rotherstein, 1985; Carmichael, 1987; Love and Brodeur, 1987; Boline et al., 1988; Cibulka et al., 1988; Rhudy et al., 1988; Herzog et al., 1989; Mootz et al., 1989; Keating et al., 1990; Mior et al., 1990).

Consequently, only anecdotal evidence exists upon which to base the use of motion palpation and, by implication, decisions regarding manipulative intervention and clinical management (Harvey and Byfield, 1991; Byfield et al., 1995). This has led to scepticism and non-acceptance in general by those outside manual practice for basing clinical judgements on unreliable indicators (Jull et al., 1988). Furthermore, in addition to questionable concordance, the validity of various palpation and motion palpation methods still remains undermined (Mootz et al., 1989; Nansel et al., 1989; Jensen et al., 1993; Hubka and Phelan, 1994; van der Wurff et al.,

2000b). This has been attributed to the fact that no valid standard or reference measure has been established against which to assess and/or confirm the accuracy of palpation findings (Harvey and Byfield, 1991). As a result previous inter-examiner agreement studies merely constitute a test of internal validity rather than a true reflection of measurement reliability (Nansel et al., 1989). Moreover, a measurement is regarded as valid or accurate if the attribute of interest is correctly measured (Wright and Feinstein, 1992). Notwithstanding, it has been reported that reliability is a necessity, but not a sufficient condition for the overall validity of a test procedure (Feinstein, 1985). Nevertheless, if a test is completely unreliable it cannot be valid (Wright and Feinstein, 1992). Therefore, in order to determine the usefulness of a diagnostic procedure such as motion palpation, full assessment of its reliability, validity and sensitivity to clinically important change (responsiveness) must take place (Haas et al., 1995a; van der Wurff et al., 2000a,b). In addition, it has been established that unreliable measurements potentially arise from three sources – the patient, the procedure and the clinician – and a complete appraisal requires consideration of all three sources (Sackett, 1980). This indicates that potential variability exists within the examination, the performance and the individual interpretation of clinical findings leading to contradictory and erroneous conclusions and questionable clinical expectations (Haas and Panzer, 1995).

SUMMARY

This chapter will address common manual examination procedures including specific psychomotor skills required during the performance of motion palpation for the purpose of segmental diagnostics. An attempt will be made to simplify and standardize a number of these skills, keeping in mind the level of undergraduate education. The book will begin with methods of locating important anatomical landmarks required by manual practitioners during both diagnostic and therapeutic application. The text will target specific fundamental psychomotor skills required during the performance of these important clinical skills. The text is constructed in such a fashion as to present these skills as basic building blocks, taking the student from accurate anatomical landmark location through to skilful performance of manual diagnostic procedures. This will include relevant skills for the various regions of the spine and pelvis plus the major joints of the upper and lower limb. Emphasis

will also be placed on the concept that clinical decisions for manipulative intervention are based upon multiple diagnostic criteria (palpation findings, pain location, tissue tenderness, asymmetry etc.) and not just one procedure in isolation.

CLINICAL PALPATION METHODS

Despite advances in diagnostic imaging and other sophisticated procedures, palpation remains a commonly used and essential skill to evaluate the neuro-musculoskeletal system within disciplines such as chiropractic, osteopathy and physical therapy (Haas and Panzer, 1995; Walker and Buchbinder, 1997; McKenzie and Taylor, 1997).

In addition to commonly used static palpatory techniques, the chiropractic profession has developed a number of dynamic forms of palpation (Gillet, 1960; Gillet and Liekens, 1969). These motion palpatory skills have been expanded and introduced as an integral foundation in college curricula (Schafer and Faye, 1989; Faye and Wiles, 1992). The American Chiropractic Association (ACA) council on technique currently defines 'palpation' as 'the application of manual pressures, through the surface of the body, to determine the shape, size, consistency, position and inherent motility of the tissues beneath' (ACA, 1988).

Types of palpation

There are two contemporary palpation techniques that are generally used to identify areas of articular and/or soft tissue dysfunction and assist in making decisions regarding manipulative intervention management (Peterson and Bergmann, 1993; Haas and Panzer, 1995).

These can be categorized as:
1. Static palpation
   a) Soft tissue
   b) Bony
2. Motion palpation
   a) Active/passive segmental range of motion
   b) Accessory motions
      - Joint play
      - End feel (end play)
      - Joint challenge (static)

Static palpation – definition

During static palpation, the patient is motionless, usually in a prone or sitting position and the examiner uses manual digital contact over osseous and soft

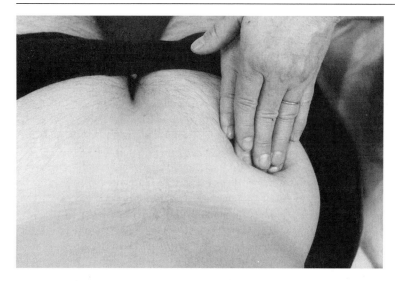

Fig. 1.1   Static palpation to detect soft tissue tone

tissues in order to detect, for example, tissue tone, tissue elasticity, tissue texture, skin temperature, assess areas of pain and tenderness and osseous alignment (Figures 1.1, 1.2, 1.3, 1.4 and 1.5). Static palpation is also employed to identify important anatomical landmarks (Figures 1.6 and 1.7a, b, c, d). Static palpation is a very basic form of tactile observation combining other visual cues. A major function of static palpation is to identify painful soft tissue structures that may be indicative of local or referred joint dysfunction. Static palpation does not assess the joint for active and/or passive accessory ranges of motion qualities. It has been determined that correct identification of anatomical landmarks and intersegmental levels is important clinically with respect to identifying the appropriate therapeutic target within the musculoskeletal system. Misidentification of exact segmental level has been

identified as a potential primary source of interobserver palpation error refuting any attempts to maintain segmental accuracy (Keating et al., 1990; McKenzie and Taylor, 1997; O' Haire and Gibbons, 2000). The issue regarding the accuracy of anatomical landmark identification, reliability and segmental specificity with respect to motion palpation will be introduced later.

Motion palpation – definition

Motion palpation has been defined as, 'palpation of the human spine in the diagnosis of muscular, discal or articular mechanical changes and used very commonly by chiropractors and osteopathic physicians to detect manipulable lesions and to evaluate patients' progress' (Alley, 1983). Furthermore, motion palpation is generally used to evaluate mus-

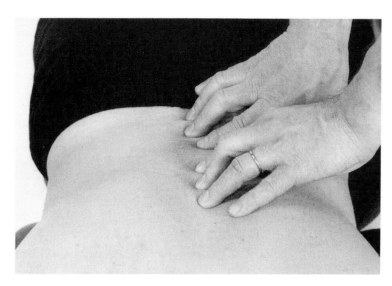

Fig. 1.2   Static palpation to detect osseous alignment

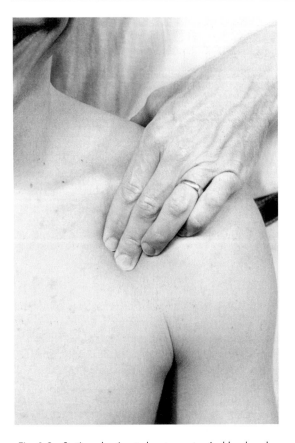

Fig. 1.3   Static palpation to locate anatomical landmarks

culoskeletal compliance, performance and assess the ability to meet these physical demands (Russell, 1983). It is a collection of manual examination skills designed to assess active passive and other accessory joint movements (Peterson and Bergman, 1993). Moreover, motion palpation is a dynamic and kinetic diagnostic procedure to determine joints in dysfunc-

tion and assess the specific direction of lost or restricted motion as an indicator prior to manipulative intervention and post-manipulative evaluation (Faye and Wiles, 1992). Motion palpation methods appraise very specific aspects of the overall active and passive ranges of motion characteristics of diarthroidial joints, which was initially conceptualized by Sandoz (1976). Panjabi (1992) redefined in terms of a spinal stabilization system and a more practical kinematic interpretation incorporating elements from both concepts was integrated by Kondracki (1996). In addition, motion palpation has been referred to as a learned kinaesthetic or 'motion' sense which is a subjective appreciation or movement arising from various proprioceptors and touch receptors (Beal, 1953; Greenman, 1989). The following represents a breakdown of the types of motion palpation.

Active/dynamic motion palpation

Dynamic motion palpation is normally carried out within the patient's active physiological range of motion to determine the quality and quantity of segmental range of motion. This is the type of motion that, by definition, can be actively performed by the individual within their normal boundaries of joint mobility. This range also includes the passive involuntary joint play motion.

The characteristics of each range of movement can be represented in a two-dimensional pattern for each individual plane of motion including flexion/extension, lateral flexion and rotation that was first interpreted by Sandoz (1976), developed by Kirkaldy-Willis and Cassidy (1985) and more recently upgraded by Peterson and Bergmann (1993)

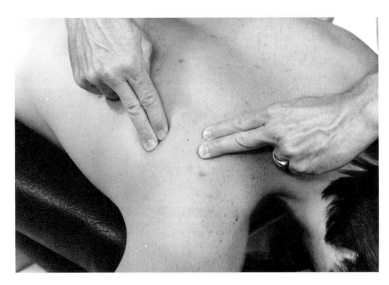

Fig. 1.4   Static palpation to assess tissue texture

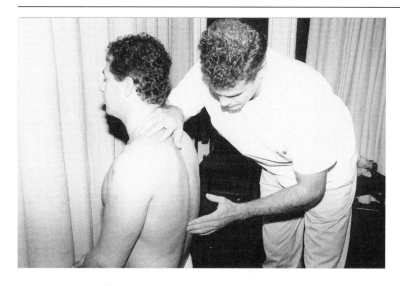

Fig. 1.5 Static palpation to identify levels of pain and tenderness

(Figure 1.8). A recent description includes a more comprehensive interpretation of all the potential types of motion within each plane of motion with all the other accessory movement characteristics. Each individual range or degree of freedom of movement demonstrates these movement characteristics, which are strongly influenced by specific joint architecture and local soft tissue morphology depending on the region of the spine. Figure 1.8 provides an overview summary of movement palpation targets relative to joint characteristics. The role of manipulation and mobilization with respect to individual influence on a specific aspect of joint motion is also described.

This two-dimensional concept of joint motion places each subdivision of the overall range of physiological motion into an order but makes no attempt

to quantify or qualify the kinematic value of the active and passive motion available. Furthermore, in vivo, viscoelastic behaviour of the spinal joint stabilizing structures behaves in a non-linear biphasic fashion as they deform under applied loads and are not represented equally (Panjabi, 1992). Active motion is produced voluntarily by the patient as a result of muscular activity and is therefore limited by many factors outside the range of passive motion. Furthermore, the examiner controls active or dynamic motion palpation procedures. The patient has no active participation. Knowledge of the average intervertebral kinematic values for each region of the spine should theoretically assist interpretation of various palpatory findings.

This individual intersegmental appreciation transcends from clinically evaluating regional or global

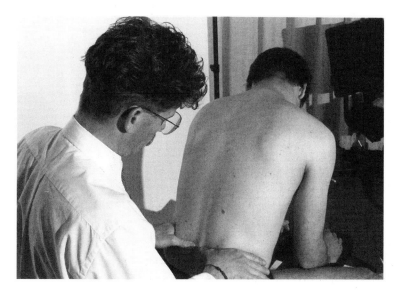

Fig. 1.6 Static palpation to identify L4 spinous process

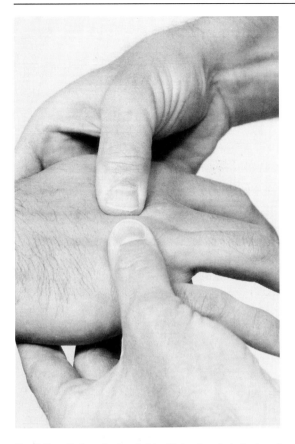

Fig. 1.7a   Static palpation to identify landmarks in the hand

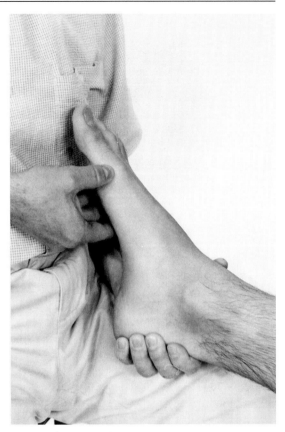

Fig. 1.7c   Static palpation to identify landmarks in the foot

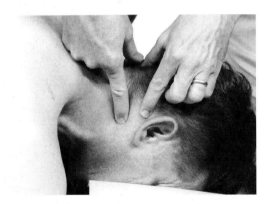

Fig. 1.7b   Static palpation to identify landmarks in the neck

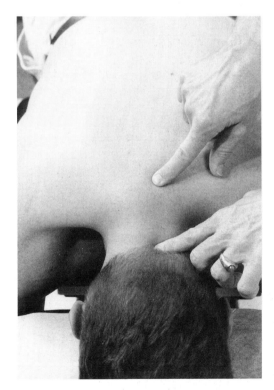

Fig. 1.7d   Static palpation to identify landmarks in the upper back

ranges of motion of the spine. Active palpation, as it was developed by Henri Gillet and developed by Len Faye and Adrian Grice, assesses the pattern of motion at each intervertebral level in any given plane of motion. The observer moves the patient fully through all the clinical ranges of motion assessing predominantly quantity and quality of movement in each range, including flexion and extension (assessing separating and approximating spinous processes) (Figures 1.9 and 1.10), lateral bending

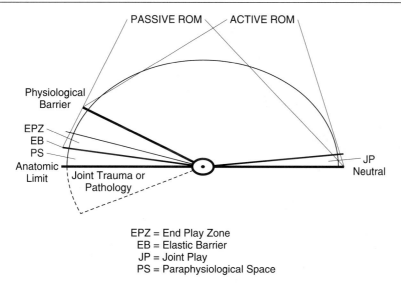

EPZ = End Play Zone
EB = Elastic Barrier
JP = Joint Play
PS = Paraphysiological Space

Fig. 1.8 The active and passive range of motion capable in one plane of a joint (adapted from Peterson and Bergmann, 1993 with permission)

(spinous to concavity) (Figure 1.11), and rotation (spinous process stairstep configuration) (Figure 1.12) contacting the spinous process or other spinal landmarks as a point of leverage. The palpator typically controls patient movements, guiding them through various directions using the free hand/fingers to palpate joint movement details throughout the entire active range of segmental motion. This type of palpation operates on the premise that normal muscle harmony must exist to ensure that

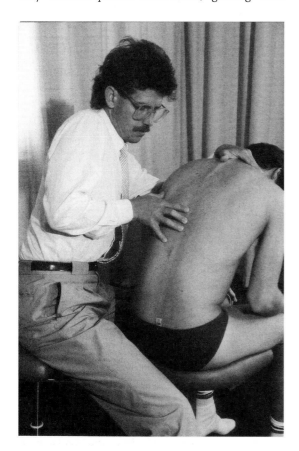

Fig. 1.9 Motion palpation in flexion

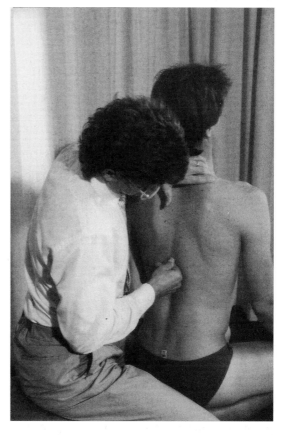

Fig. 1.10 Motion palpation in extension

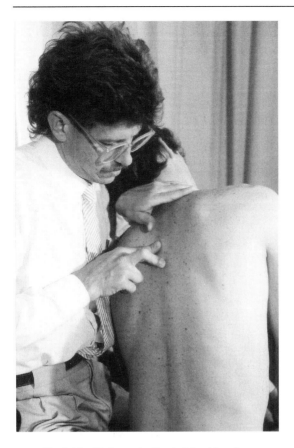

Fig. 1.11   Motion palpation in lateral bending

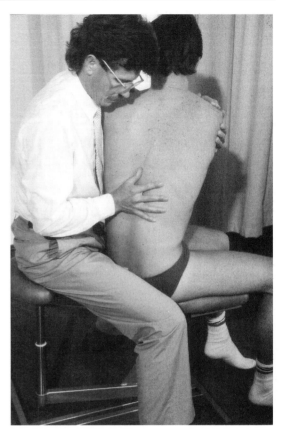

Fig. 1.12   Motion palpation in rotation

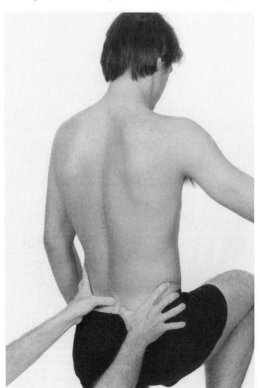

Fig. 1.13   Motion palpation of the sacroiliac joints

normal spinal motion takes place (Fligg, 1984). This is particularly evident during motion palpation examination of the sacroiliac joints (Figure 1.13). By evaluating the segmental kinematic pattern of motion in all planes, the observer can determine motion segment balance and function. Any abnormalities detected may help establish a palpatory diagnosis of joint dysfunction and guide subsequent manipulative intervention (Schafer and Faye, 1989). There are many problems with this assessment, due mainly to the fact that the palpator is attempting to assess extremely small kinematic ranges of motion, not to mention the range of biological variation that exists within the general population. This may partially explain why such poor inter-observer reliability has been recorded for motion palpation skills. This will be discussed in greater detail later in the chapter.

Passive accessory palpation

Passive motion or accessory joint movements are described as small normal involuntary movements (Mennell, 1960, 1964). This type of accessory motion can exceed the patient's voluntary active range of motion and is normally assessed by the

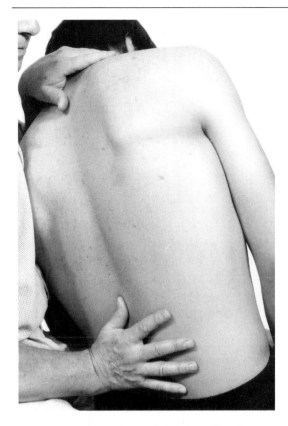

Fig. 1.14a   End play analysis in lateral bending

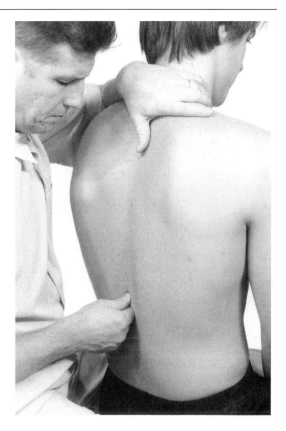

Fig. 1.14b   End play analysis in extension

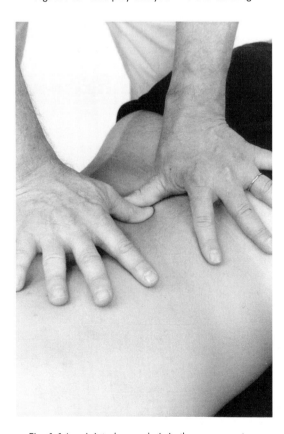

Fig. 1.14c   Joint play analysis in the prone posture

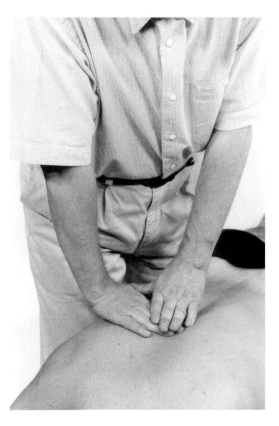

Fig. 1.14d   Joint play analysis in the prone posture

examiner at the end of the passive range of spinal joint motion at the elastic barrier of the joint and is known as *end play* or *end feel* in the sitting weight-bearing posture (Figure1.14a, b) and *joint play* or *challenge* in the prone non-weight-bearing position (Figure 1.14c, d) (Peterson and Bergmann, 1993). End play qualitatively assesses the progressive resistance through the end play zone at the end of passive joint movement (ACA Council on Technic, 1988). Refer to Figure 1.8 for the relative position of each specific motion type and its position in the overall range of motion. Here the assessor assesses the joint at the end of the passive range of motion. This motion is often described as the natural 'give' and 'spring' associated with normally functioning diarthroidial joints and related soft tissues. If clinically significant, this will have a very hard end feel and is usually accompanied by associated tenderness. This 'give' has recently been referred to as the elastic zone (EZ), which is defined as a progressive increase in ligamentous stiffness towards the end of normal joint range of motion and related to overall joint stability (Panjabi, 1992; Kondracki, 1996) (Figure 1.15). Figure 1.15 illustrates the inherent viscoelasticity of synovial joints and the non-linearity behaviour

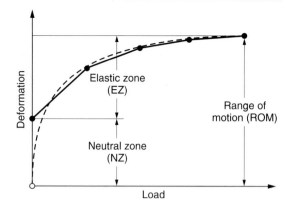

Fig. 1.15 Load deformation characteristics of a joint including the neutral zone (NZ) of high flexibility and elastic zone (EZ) of increased stiffness (adapted from Kondracki, 1996 with permission)

exhibited during load deformation. This more recent concept closely parallels the active, passive, elastic barrier motion characteristics schematically illustrated in Figure 1.8 and will be discussed later in more detail under kinematics and motion palpation. This is characteristically described in detail for the spinal joints but can be extrapolated to assess the inherent joint play of the major extremity joints that are also described in this text and are important from a clinical perspective particularly in sports-related injuries (Figure 1.16a,b).

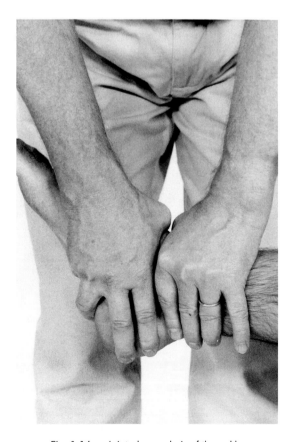

Fig. 1.16a Joint play analysis of the ankle

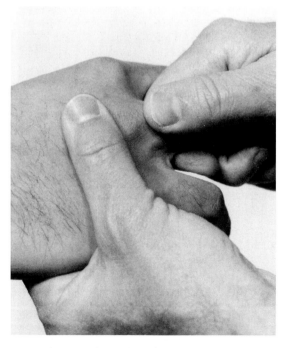

Fig. 1.16b Joint play analysis of the metacarpalphalangeal joint

A number of corresponding examination procedures have been developed to assess these joint motion characteristics including joint play (Mennell, 1960), end feel (Mennell, 1960; Cyriax, 1975; Kessler, 1983; Gillet and Liekens, 1969; Fligg, 1984; Faye and Wiles, 1992), joint challenge (Fligg, 1984) and end play (Peterson and Bergmann, 1993). Keep an eye on Figure 1.8 for terminology and specific range of motion and a description later in the text. The major differences are between joint play (joint challenge) and end play (end feel). These procedures will be described in detail in the subsequent chapters of the book for all areas of the spine and pelvis.

Joint play originally developed out of a need to test for the involuntary movements of diarthroidial joints and, in this case, including the extremity articulations and was extrapolated to include the zygapophyseal joints of the spinal column (Mennell, 1960, 1964). It was established that clinically these involuntary movements must exist in order that voluntary movements should take place. This suggests that the presence of both normal active (voluntary) and passive (involuntary) movements are a prerequisite for normal biomechanical joint function. In addition to the normal active and passive ranges of motion, there are accessory motions characteristic of diarthroidial joints which are reflected in the inherent viscoelastic properties and are also referred to as end play (feel) and joint play (Mennell, 1960; Schafer and Faye, 1989; Bergmann and Peterson, 1995).

In other words, total joint motion is the sum of the voluntary range of movement (active) plus an additional involuntary range (passive) which includes the accessory movements (joint play and end play) (see Figure 1.8). Accessory movements occur because normal joint surfaces do not appose tightly. The capsule of the joint must allow some extra play or give for full motion to occur. Movement beyond the active range, including accessory movements, cannot be produced by muscle contraction, however, voluntary motion is influenced by normal accessory mechanics (Schafer and Faye, 1989). These accessory and passive movements are necessary for full painless function of the joint as well as complete voluntary range of motion (Magee, 1987).

Accessory joint movements are assessed predominantly by joint play and end feel (play) procedures (Mennell, 1960; Schafer and Faye, 1989; Faye and Wiles, 1992; Peterson and Bergmann, 1993). Joint play movements are a qualitative evaluation of the joint's resistance to induced movement from the

neutral or loose-packed non-weight-bearing position (see Figure 1.14b) (Magee, 1987; Peterson and Bergmann, 1993). These joint play movements are contained within the confines of the synovial joint capsule (Mennell, 1990). In quantifiable terms, it has been suggested that the extent of any joint play movement in any synovial joint is less than 5 mm in any plane from a neutral position (Mennell, 1991). Movement beyond the elastic barrier into the paraphysiological space has been recorded in the 3–5 mm range during axial distraction at the carpometacarpophalangeal joint (Sandoz, 1976). This does give some indication of the extremely small amount of movement elicited during these palpatory methods and how differences in interpretation are possible.

End play accessory movements, on the other hand are distinctly different. End play is designated as joint play challenge administered at the end range of joint motion just prior to elastic barrier at the physiological limit of joint motion (see Figure 1.14a) (Sandoz, 1976; Schafer and Faye, 1989; Peterson and Bergmann, 1993) (Figure 1.8). This is usually assessed in the close-packed weight-bearing position of the joint and mainly at the spinal intersegmental level. This differentiation fits naturally into the biphasic non-linear behaviour of joint motion proposed by Panjabi (1992) and eloquently translated into clinical perspective by Kondracki (1996).

Therefore, the load-deformation spinal stability concepts of NZ and EZ (see Figure 1.15) are fully compatible with the types of joint motion presented in Figure 1.8 to describe various motion palpation assessment procedures as follows:

This may provide insight into the possible effects

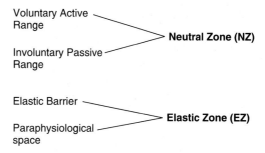

of spinal manipulation on these specific characteristics of joint mobility (Cassidy et al., 1993).

In conclusion

Motion palpation may be defined as both a quantitative and qualitative form of joint assessment as defined by the boundaries and characteristics of joint motion (Alley, 1983). This brief description of motion palpation terminology, various assessment differences and similarities relating to the overall joint mobility characteristics are integral to the objectives of this study and the discussion regarding procedural and terminology standardization.

KINEMATICS AND MOTION PALPATION

An in-depth and thorough knowledge of spinal bio-mechanics, especially kinematics, is essential to the understanding of the clinical analysis, diagnostics and treatment of various spinal syndromes. This begins with a fundamental understanding of the ter-minology used in kinematics.

Kinematics vs Kinetics

Kinematics is that branch of mechanics that is concerned with the kinds and amounts of motion rigid bodies undergo, without concern for the forces that are responsible for the motion (Galley and Forster, 1987). Kinematics takes into account important parameters, such as displacement, velocity, acceleration and time (White and Panjabi, 1990). Kinetics, on the other hand, is concerned with the forces that are responsible for the motion or any changes in the motion.

Right-handed cartesian coordinate system

This is a rectangular coordinate system most preferred for defining the position and motion of rigid bodies in space. This system is illustrated in three dimensions which permits a three-dimensional description of motion of an object.

Three axes, x, y, and z (Figure 1.17a,b) or sagittal, coronal and horizontal planes (Figure 1.18) define the coordinate system. This system permits description of a motion unit (motor unit, functional spinal unit) which consists of two contiguous vertebrae with their intervening soft tissues. Motion is described in terms of movement of the upper vertebra on the subadjacent vertebra. Each vertebra has six degrees of freedom: rotation about and translation along a transverse, sagittal and a longitudinal axis (Norkin and Levangie, 1992). The motion of the spine as a whole and each individual motion unit produced during flexion, extension, lateral flexion and axial rotation is a complex combined motion resulting from simultaneous rotation and translation (Lindh, 1989).

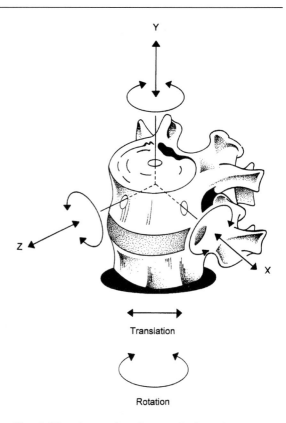

Fig. 1.17a A complete intervertebral motion segment including the x, y, z, coordinate axes

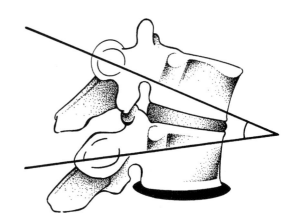

Fig. 1.17b A motion segment rotating around the x-axis

Types of motion

A) *Rotation* (rotary, angular motion) involves motion of a spinal motion unit in a curved path, about or around a fixed axis. A spinning or angular displacement of an object occurs around an axis. The axis may be located within an object, or outside, some distance from the moving object (Figure 1.17a).

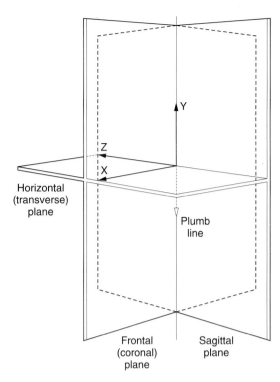

Fig. 1.18 The various axes and planes used to describe various kinematic motion behaviour

B) *Translation* (translatory motion) occurs when the motion of a spinal motion unit is in a straight line in that all points on the object move in parallel paths, through the same distance, at the same time. This is a linear translation. Sliding and gliding are also used interchangeably to describe translation (Figure 1.17a).

Degrees of freedom

When a rigid body, for example a spinal motion unit, translates back and forth along an axis, or rotates back and forth around an axis, the object is said to exhibit one degree of freedom. Since a vertebra can exhibit translation along each of the three main axes (x, y, z) and rotation around each of the same axes, it possesses six degrees of freedom (White and Panjabi, 1990). Coupled motion or coupling occurs when translation or rotation take place along or around two different axes simultaneously. For example, cervical and lumbar horizontal plane rotation (y-axis rotation) is coupled with coronal plane rotation (z-axis rotation). Spinal motion is generally multiplanar and qualitatively described using the system.

On the other hand, paradoxical motion can be associated with a dysfunctional motion segment or instability and occurs when a typical motion is expected but, in fact, the opposite motion is described (Grice, 1979). For example, during cervical spine flexion, there should be an anterior translation (+ z-axis translation), however, a paradoxical posterior translation (z-axis translation) may occur leading to possible pathophysiological changes to the soft tissue holding elements at the motion segment. Of important note are the effects of abnormal or excessive spinal motion unit kinematic activity as a result of holding element laxity that would lead to clinical instability. Such instability may produce abnormal coupling, abnormal patterns of motion and irregular instantaneous axes of rotation further comprising motion unit integrity (Panjabi and White, 1990). It is this intersegmental type of motion that manual therapists are attempting to assess during various motion palpation examinations of the spine.

More recently, Panjabi (1992) proposed that *in vivo* viscoelastic behaviour is non-linear and biphasic with respect to spinal stability which allows for greater movement within the neutral position, but progressively limits motion towards the end of this range. This area of relative ligamentous laxity has been defined as the neutral zone (NZ) and the region of increasing ligamentous stiffness is known as the elastic zone (EZ) (Panjabi, 1992). It has been proposed that an increase in the NZ represents instability and that a reduction in this region of low bending moment (NZ) would characterize a spinal fixation (Kondracki, 1996). This perceived tissue resistance that is reportedly detected during motion palpation is most likely an appreciation of the EZ sooner than appreciated, with a reduction in the overall neutral range (NZ) constituting a unique joint fixation and the clinical implications represent an update of the earlier 'elastic barrier' and paraphysiological space concepts presented by Sandoz (1976) in relation to the effects of chiropractic manipulation on joint mechanics. Therefore, it would be an advantage clinically to have some knowledge of the normal values of corresponding spinal motion segments both from a diagnostic and therapeutic perspective (Kondracki, 1996).

Knowledge of the normal kinematics at various levels and, more importantly, the dominant plane of motion could be invaluable to the clinician in identifying a number of clinical abnormalities which may benefit from manipulative intervention. The coupling patterns of the lower cervical spine have been established (Lysell, 1969; Panjabi et al., 1986; Moroney et al., 1988). However, coupling in the lumbar spine remains controversial, particularly the association between axial rotation and lateral bending (Pope et al., 1977; Stokes et al., 1981). Knowledge of these coupling patterns is crucial as motion palpation skills are some of the most difficult to master for students of chiropractic (Kondracki, 1996). Mental imaging and an understanding of the positive biomechanical therapeutic outcomes has been shown to enhance psychomotor skills acquisition (Byfield, 1996). Calls for tighter educational controls and professional standardization of motion palpation methods has been proclaimed by many authors (Love and Brodeur, 1987; Panzer, 1992). This concept will be presented in more depth in Chapter 3 dealing with quantifying palpation parameters.

CLINICAL CONSIDERATIONS AND KINEMATICS

Gonella et al. (1982) and Keating et al. (1990) found poor inter-examiner reliability specifically for active motion palpation methods of the lumbar spine. This is not particularly surprising when considering the complex kinematic behaviour of the lumbar motion segments. Rotation, for example, is limited to 1–2 degrees at most, which is potentially very difficult to detect from a palpation and kinaesthetic perspective (Bogduk and Twomey, 1987; White and Panjabi, 1990). However, in this instance the perception of movement is often more important than the degree of movement, which would be subject to practitioner interpretation and contribute to poor reliability. Since the overall range of kinematic behaviour at an intersegmental level is so small, particularly in the lumbar spine, it may simply be enough to indicate that motion exists or does not from a qualitative rather than a quantitative point of view.

Yamamota et al. (1989) established kinematic magnitudes of 1.5–2.6 degrees of axial rotation in the lumbar spine with least motion at the L5/S1 motion segment. To the authors' knowledge, no one to date has determined what the threshold for detection of small angular movements actually is in quantitative terms. The ability to detect this angular displacement may be an important clinical skill, particularly when examiners may be capable of detecting such small ranges of motion described by the lumbar intervertebral joints. Nonetheless, there is about 5 degrees of lateral bending at each lumbar segment (White and Panjabi, 1990). This amount of movement is conceivably more palpable, remembering that this movement is of a coupled nature which would be included in rotation. The largest active range of movement takes place in the sagittal

plane during flexion and extension (sagittal rotation). This equates to about 14 degrees on average for each motion segment over a full range of flexion/extension, with greater flexion than extension at each level (White and Panjabi, 1990). The largest range is in the lower lumbar motion segments, 10.1 degrees for L1/L2 to 17.8 degrees for L5/S1 (Yamamota et al., 1989). This amount of angular movement could conceivably be palpable even though there has been no experimental evidence to the contrary. The findings of this study demonstrated that posture and intervertebral level are two important factors in determining the magnitude and characteristics of both the main and coupled motions in the lumbar spine (Yamamota et al., 1989). Therefore, common palpation postures (sitting, supine, prone) could significantly influence the type and nature of movement in the lumbar spine and influence palpation outcome.

None of the active palpation studies to date have actually divided the motion segments into specific directional fixations (rotation, lateral bending or flexion/extension) or compared these with the known kinematic characteristics for that region of the spine. The assumption that all six ranges of motion at each segment should be examined may be clinically unnecessary, as each region of the spine has quite distinct movement patterns and kinematic characteristics (White and Panjabi, 1990). This approach needs to be modified to permit better standardization of motion palpation skills, both from a research and educational point of view.

Summary

Current evidence fails to support the use of motion palpation methods alone for the determination of joint dysfunction including decisions regarding the target site for manipulative intervention. There is also lack of acceptable consensus in the chiropractic profession as to the best methods of spinal palpation (Hubka, 1994). This represents an area of investigation that could lead to standardized experimental protocols that would permit comparison of results in future reliability and validity studies.

Furthermore, the need to evaluate seriously individual diagnostic methods such as motion palpation as part of an integrated multidimensional biomechanical clinical examination is supported by its well documented widespread use (Gitelman, 1980; Kirkaldy-Willis, 1988). It would therefore appear sensible to expect that provision of a standardized palpatory procedure for the spine could improve reliability methodology for future studies.

INTERVERTEBRAL JOINT FIXATION OR INTERSEGMENTAL RESTRICTION – DEFINITION

Following from motion palpation, the assessment of normal arises from the identification of abnormal or restricted motion. The concept of joint fixation has played a significant part in the biomechanical paradigm of the chiropractic profession for many years (Gillet, 1960; Gillet and Liekens, 1969; Schafer and Faye, 1989; Bergmann and Peterson, 1995).

A joint fixation is defined as a spinal and/or extraspinal articular mobility restriction (Schafer and Faye, 1989). A fixation refers to any physical, functional or psychological mechanism that produces a loss of segmental mobility within its normal physiological range of motion (Schafer and Faye, 1989). Furthermore, a fixation is a clinical entity whereby a joint articulation has become temporarily immobilized in a phase of normal physiological movement pattern (Figure 1.8). It has become synonymous with the manipulable lesion from a clinical point of view and has been labelled as that entity that is actively identified and differentiated during motion palpation procedures before and after therapeutic application (Gitelman, 1980; Grice, 1980). Motion palpation methods were developed to detect restricted articular motion or excess mobility in order to administer the appropriate manipulative therapy (Gillet, 1960). These areas of joint dysfunction, which are typically defined as disturbances of joint function without structural change, affect both quality and range of motion and are diagnosed with the aid of motion palpation (Peterson, 1993).

It is not the intent of this chapter to engage in a discussion of the formidable task of evaluating primary joint dysfunction. It is, however, pivotal at this stage to indicate that a diagnosis of primary joint dysfunction is difficult to establish due to the limited understanding of the pathomechanics and pathophysiology of this clinical entity (Acker et al., 1990; Triano, 1990; Liebenson, 1992).

Furthermore, no evidence of structural alteration exists and validated criteria for detecting joint dysfunction are currently not available (Harvey and Byfield, 1991; Peterson, 1993). This very issue constitutes one of the primary objectives of this study which focuses on validating a reference measure against which to assess motion palpation skills. The reliability and validity of motion palpation procedures will be presented in the next section of this review.

MOTION PALPATION RELIABILITY AND VALIDITY STUDIES

More than 90 research articles have appeared in the peer reviewed chiropractic literature concerning the reliability and validity of various clinical procedures (Haas, 1991a; Haas and Panzer, 1995). Close to 30 research papers have been published investigating the inter- and intra-examiner reliability of various palpation procedures (Haas, 1991a). A number of studies have been published since 1991, but in total, 22 studies have reported original data on the reliability of motion palpation (Wiles, 1980; DeBoer et al., 1985; Potter and Rothstein, 1985; Mior et al., 1984; Bergstrom and Courtis, 1986; Carmichael, 1987; Love and Brodeur, 1987; Boline et al., 1988; Nansel and Jansen, 1988; Rhudy et al., 1988; Herzog et al., 1989; LeBoeuf et al., 1989; Mootz et al., 1989; Nansel et al., 1989; Keating et al., 1990; Mior et al., 1990; Paydar et al., 1994; Haas et al., 1995a; Tuchin et al., 1996; Hawk et al., 1999; Toussaint et al., 1999; French et al., 2000). It was concluded that there have been very few well designed studies conducted to draw any definitive conclusions concerning the consistency of motion palpation methods (Haas, 1991a; Troyanovich et al., 1998; van der Wurff et al., 2000 a, b).

In addition, 12 review articles have been published scrutinizing motion palpation reliability studies with respect to methodological design, statistical appropriateness and conclusions drawn (Alley, 1983; Russell, 1983; Banks and Willis, 1988; Dishman, 1988; Keating, 1988a, 1989a; Haas, 1991a; Breen, 1992; Panzer, 1992; Walker, 1996; Hersboek and Lebouef-Yde, 2000; van der Wurff et al., 2000a). Most, if not all studies demonstrated poor inter-examiner reliability (average study kappa = 0.00–0.15) and moderate intra-examiner concordance (average study kappa = 0.45 – 0.53) (Haas, 1991a; Haas and Panzer, 1995; Haas et al., 1995b).

A number of authors have reviewed various palpation techniques, providing definitions and procedural distinctions for specific palpatory techniques (Alley, 1983; Russell, 1983). Lack of palpatory standardization has been identified as a potential confounding factor in a number of reliability trials as well as a number of methodological design flaws (Alley, 1983; Keating, 1989a; Haas, 1991a, b). Keating (1989a) systematically reviewed the methodology of seven palpation reliability studies concerning motion palpation of the thoracolumbar spine with respect to the type of palpation, examiners and their qualifications, characteristics of the sample, spinal level examined, unit of measurement, statistical evaluation and findings, and conclusions drawn. This analysis did not provide strong evidence of the inter-examiner reliability of lumbar motion palpation that would justify any strong claims (Keating, 1989a).

These conclusions were echoed by a number of other authors reviewing additional trials post 1989 (Haas, 1991a; Breen, 1992; Panzer, 1992; Walker 1996; van der Wurff, 2000a, b). van der Wurff (2000a) reviewed six studies that evaluated sacroiliac motion palpation. The methodology review included three criteria: the study population, the test procedures, the test results. In two of the studies, sacroiliac motion palpation was shown to be reliable. However, these studies demonstrated low methodological scores and therefore were considered to be flawed. This led the authors to conclude that it would be difficult to envisage an improvement in results even with methodological upgrading. Panzer (1992) analysed ten lumbar palpation reliability studies in a similiar fashion to Keating (1989a) and concluded that poor inter-examiner and moderate intra-examiner reliability was generally reported. A number of potential sources of error were cited in these studies, including inadequate experience of the examiners, misidentification of exact segmental level, examiner fatigue, delay between palpation sessions, inadequate standardization and an over-emphasis on clinically insignificant findings (Panzer, 1992). Particular importance was placed upon the misuse and inappropriate statistical analysis which lacked inclusion of chance corrected inferential statistics (kappa), resulting in misinterpretation of overall test concordance (Haas, 1991b; Keating, 1992). Keating (1989a) stated emphatically that motion palpation should be used on a limited basis as its usefulness, reliability and validity are undetermined. This statement should be interpreted with caution as this only refers to the objectivity of a single evaluative tool being scrutinized in isolation from other clinical procedures which would normally constitute a more comprehensive clinical assessment protocol.

Of the 22 motion palpation reliability studies published to date:

- Six concern cervical spine palpation (DeBoer et al., 1985; Mior et al., 1985; Nansel and Jansen, 1988; Rhudy et al., 1988; Nansel et al., 1989; Tuchin et al., 1996)
- Three concern thoracic spine palpation (Nansel and Jansen, 1988; Rhudy et al., 1988; Haas et al., 1995a)

- Eight concern lumbar spine palpation (Bergstrom and Courtis, 1986; Love and Brodeur, 1987; Boline et al., 1988; Rhudy et al., 1988; Nansel and Jansen, 1988; LeBoeuf et al., 1989; Mootz et al., 1989; Keating et al., 1990; Hawk et al., 1999; French et al., 2000).
- Nine concern sacroiliac joint palpation (Wiles, 1980; Carmichael, 1987; Nansel and Jansen, 1988; Herzog et al., 1989; LeBeouf et al., 1989; Mior et al., 1990; Paydar et al., 1994; Toussaint et al., 1999; French et al., 2000).

A number of these studies have demonstrated good experimental protocol including appropriate statistical application and compatible conclusions (Mior et al.,1984; Love and Brodeur, 1987; Mootz et al., 1989; Keating et al., 1990; Mior et al., 1990). The following is a synopsis of these and a few selected studies published outside the chiropractic profession for comparison. It should be noted that care was taken not to generalize results from other professional investigations due to contrasting teaching and palpation methods.

Reliability studies

Gonella et al. (1982) assessed the reliability of passive motion palpation of five physiotherapists in the lumbar spine, which involved both normal and blindfolded assessments using palpatory techniques described by Kaltenborn and Lindahl (1969). The researchers found no significant inter-therapist reliability, but acceptable intra-therapist concordance. No inferential statistical analysis was provided, therefore any definitive conclusions were speculative due to a methodologically weak experimental design.

An intra- and inter-examiner study investigating the reliability of passive motion palpation in the upper cervical spine revealed fair intra-observer agreement, but no significant inter-observer agreement beyond chance (Mior et al., 1984). A similar study incorporating both static and passive motion palpation to identify tenderness, altered tissue structure and joint fixation in the cervical spine found strong intra- and inter-examiner reliability at C6 and C7 spinal levels only, but lacked any concordance at the C2–C5 levels, concluding that the examiners may have responded to different palpatory clues (DeBoer et al., 1985).

These conclusions were echoed in a later study investigating end range joint play reliability during lateral flexion of the mid to lower cervical spine (Nansel et al., 1989). It was concluded that the inter-examiner agreement rates were not significantly different from those expected by chance alone.

Significant reproducibility was reported between examiners when locating hypomobile segments at the thoracolumbar spine (Love and Brodeur, 1987). However, when the data were re-evaluated, it was identified that the use of the Pearson product moment correlation coefficient was improperly applied, leading to the conclusion there was no agreement beyond chance for the data set analysed (Keating, 1989a). A screening procedure was employed in this study which typically identifies mulitsegmental regions rather than a segment by segment appraisal, suggesting that sensitivity would be of greater importance than specificity. This was regarded as an experimental flaw (Keating, 1988b). This study was also criticized for employing examiners with limited experience (Belski, 1988).

An inter-examiner reliability study of passive motion palpation to detect intersegmental restrictions and static palpation for pain and muscle tension detection in the lumbar spine found weak, but statistically significant agreement for fixations and muscle tension only at T12/L1 and the L3/4 intervertebral levels (Boline et al., 1988). When asymptomatic individuals were excluded, weak concordance for intersegmental restrictions was noted at T12/L1 and L3/4 and much stronger concordance for pain was found at L2/L3 and L3/L4. No agreement beyond chance was found in the lower lumbar spine.

The reliability of two experienced chiropractors using passive palpation techniques to locate spinal fixations in the lumbar spine established only moderate test-retest agreement beyond chance at L1/L2, minimal reliability at L4/L5, and no significant agreement between examiners in the mid-lumbar spine (Mootz et al., 1989). In fact, inter-examiner agreement for all segments was poor (kappa 0.17), providing no support for the inter-examiner reliability of passive motion palpation to detect fixations in the lumbar spine.

Keating et al. (1990) investigated the reliability of different examination procedures, including visual observation, skin temperature, palpation for osseous and soft tissue pain, muscle tension, misalignment palpation and active passive palpation. They found marginal to good agreement beyond chance for palpatory pain over osseous structures and in paraspinal soft tissues. They found little significance between examiners for active and passive motion palpation, muscle tension and misalignment palpation. This study, similar to others, did not define the experimental palpation procedure. Their results suggested

that subjective procedures (pain location) may be among the more reliable diagnostic observations. Experimental designs incorporating a multidimensional diagnostic approach is a clear diversion from the more traditional concordance investigation of individual skills seen in the literature to date.

Significant correlation between examiners assessing sacroiliac joint mobility concluded that these motion palpation tests had a high specificity and low sensitivity (Wiles, 1980). Potter and Rothstein (1985), on the other hand, found that inter-tester reliability of sacroiliac joint dysfunction was generally poor, demonstrating 50% agreement or less.

Yet, in another study, only fair intra-examiner concordance and minimal agreement was found between examiners employing standardized sacroiliac motion palpation tests (Carmichael, 1987). Haas (1991a) concluded that the study was not supported by appropriate inferential statistics for that particular experimental design and data set. Similarly, a different research team investigating consistency of the same sacroiliac palpatory methods also established statistically significant intra-examiner reliability (Herzog et al., 1989). Greater experience in this particular study appeared to lower intra-observer agreement scores. These results contradict the conclusions of Mior et al. (1990), who argued that clinical experience and teaching method had little effect on the outcome of palpation agreement rates for sacroiliac joint palpation diagnosis. The latter research team came to the conclusion that clinicians follow a set of criteria and standards that are very difficult to identify and control when incorporated into informal decision making systems. The reliability of performing sacroiliac motion palpation by chiropractic interns was compared with their results prior to and following one year of clinical experience (Mior et al., 1990). Kappa values for the interns ranged from 0.00 to 0.30, with no significant differences noted at the end of one year of clinical experience. Similar views were expressed by (Rhudy et al., 1988) who investigated spinal assessment skills including motion palpation and full spine radiographs. They concluded that inter-examiner/inter-technique analysis overall lacked consistency and that clinical judgements made by individual chiropractors were probably based more on other unidentified impressions than on the information derived from the procedures themselves.

Recently, specific end play restriction palpation in the seated position in the thoracic spine demonstrated poor inter-examiner concordance (k = 0.14) and only moderate test-retest consistency (k = 0.55 and 0.43 for two examiners) (Haas et al., 1995a). These findings matched in most previous studies for other regions of the spine.

Alternatively, individual examiners have been allowed to use their own discretion, when choosing which motion palpation technique to utilize (French et al., 2000). This may have prevented any error associated with the learning of new or different psychomotor skills. Nevertheless, the outcomes of the results were only able to demonstrate fair inter-examiner agreement when pooled across all spinal joints.

A number of palpation studies have used a custom motion palpation stool which offers both a standard palpation format, ease of palpation and comfort to the patient (Mootz et al., 1989; Keating et al., 1990). A standard scanning technique to locate the area of greatest hypomobility followed by specific palpating procedures to determine the exact direction of joint play loss has been introduced effectively (Love and Brodeur, 1987; Boline et al., 1988). All examiners agreed upon the procedure to be used and what was expected during palpation sessions, indicating some degree of study standardization. They did not, however, state clearly whether there was specific and organized rehearsal time prior to the onset of the palpation sessions.

Other studies included a pre-study rehearsal time as part of the methodological design (Love and Brodeur, 1987; Boline et al., 1988; Mootz et al., 1989). Rehearsal time should be a standard protocol to ensure that all observers are performing the same standard palpation tests regardless of training and experience. Significant differences in methodological procedures have been reported to reduce any opportunity to compare the results of similar studies (Koran, 1975b). Moreover, one study was able to demonstrate slightly improved reliability when inter-examiner agreement was assessed between colleagues who had worked together for many years (Strender et al., 1997).

Finally, the feasibility of developing an objective and multidimensional rating system for the detection of spinal segmental abnormalities has been investigated (Keating et al., 1990). This research team looked at the various clinical methods of evaluating for the presence of a subluxation complex/manipulable lesion in both symptomatic and asymptomatic patients. The reliability of eight non-invasive segmental strategies including detecting pain over bony landmarks, pain in the surrounding soft tissue, muscle tension, temperature, active and passive motion palpation were investigated as individual and combined protocols. Their results showed good and significant concordance for pain on palpation over osseous structures, as was the detection of soft tissue pain at segmental levels. Their conclusions suggested that the more subjective findings of pain may be among the most reliable of conservative spinal observations. Significant correlation was found when positive findings for the eight segmental dimensions at each lumbar level were summed to form a composite joint abnormality index. This study also suggests that reliability is most likely a combined phenomenon that upon reflection makes investigation of single evaluation tools in isolation an unrealistic proposition. The question of combined reliability is still unanswered at this point. It is still unclear whether overall reliability is enhanced in conjunction with other diagnostic parameters (Keating et al., 1990; Bergmann and Peterson, 1995).

Validity studies

In an attempt to determine the construct validity of end-play palpation, Haas et al. (1995b) challenged the theoretical construct that examiners are capable of discerning improvement in thoracic spine joint restriction following manipulative intervention. In the absence of an acceptable 'internal' standard against which to measure segmental mobility changes, these researchers utilized an external, but not absolute standard, spinal manipulation and demonstrated that chiropractors are capable of detecting changes in end-play restriction in human subjects (Haas et al., 1995b).

Support for the concurrent validity of motion palpation of the cervical spine as a single diagnostic application has received support (Jull et al., 1988). Complete agreement (100% sensitivity) was established between a palpator's findings of motion dysfunction at one cervical intervertebral segment compared with a diagnostic facet block at the same level. This study has been criticized as the experimental protocol was a combined index of both pain and motion restriction which ultimately did not evaluate motion palpation alone as a single clinical tool (Haas et al., 1995b). It could be argued that the Jull et al. (1988) study confirmed that palpation for cervical spine tenderness over osseous structures is a highly reliable examination tool which has been demonstrated in later trials (Keating et al., 1990; Boline et al., 1993; Hubka and Phelan, 1994). Moreover, investigating the reliability of a single evaluative tool has recently been criticized as it is out of context with normal clinical examination procedures which are normally more comprehensive in nature (Keating et al., 1990; Haas, 1991c; Boline et al., 1993).

Currently there are no studies concerning the trial validity of motion palpation as most controlled trials investigating spinal manipulation have failed to monitor spinal segmental motion, focusing instead on general clinical outcomes (Keating, 1988c). In addition, studies of the concurrent validity of motion palpation have also been sparse and unsatisfactory (DeBoer et al., 1985).

Summary

A number of authors have critically reviewed the various reliability studies published to date regarding palpation and other related clinical procedures. Their conclusions consistently reported that many trials failed to address procedural objectivity due to poor experimental design and/or inappropriate statistical analysis (Haas, 1991a; Panzer, 1992; Haas and Panzer, 1995). Of the studies that adhered to a more stringent experimental protocol, only marginal concordance at best has been demonstrated. Of the approximately 50 studies reviewed, only 10 were determined to have properly supported conclusions, while 50% of the studies were based upon inappropriate conclusions or inconclusive statistical analyses. Although several measurement strategies deserve replication, the current literature demonstrates only marginal reliability based on a limited number of examiners of varying experience and an over reliance on results gathered from asymptomatic subjects. We would now like to discuss examiner experience followed by statistical considerations, kinematics and motion palpation and the specificity assumption of regarding joint manipulation.

SEGMENTAL IDENTIFICATION AND SPECIFICITY ASSUMPTION

Tissue movement on repeated palpation sessions and consistent segmental identification between examiners present inherent problems experimentally (Burton et al., 1990). It has also been documented that misidentification of segmental level is a common source of examiner error suggesting some measure of inaccuracy in static palpation landmark location skills (Keating et al., 1990). This could be the result of tissue movement, recording errors, and

examiner bias and could pose potential problems when palpatory findings are compared from one palpating posture to another (Byfield and Humphreys, 1992). Effectively blinding observers on successive palpation sessions is a key element when conducting studies evaluating procedural reliability. Blindfolding the palpator or placing a cover over the spine would interrupt normal clinical protocols. Recording palpation findings on familiar proforma would also reduce a potential source of error.

A marker pen visible under ultraviolet light (UV) has been shown to be a useful blinding technique for examining palpatory reliability (Burton et al., 1990; Byfield and Humphreys, 1992; Simmonds and Kumar, 1993; McKenzie and Taylor, 1997; Downey et al., 1999). It was found that this type of marking system was very successful in blinding repeated palpation observations in a typical clinical setting. This simulated the use of an ordinary pen which many practitioners use to identify the level of dysfunction when examining and treating patients. Blindfolding an observer eliminates very important visual cues which form part of the set for standards used by individual clinicians when making a decision as to whether a fixation is present or not (Mior et al., 1990). Using 'invisible' marks that can be illuminated later eliminates clinicians having to identify the segmental level. This maintains methodological consistency and eliminates recording errors. Furthermore, clinical indicators such as provocation pain over bony landmarks (spinous process) and paravertebral soft tissues once considered highly subjective, have been demonstrated to be a more reliable clinical procedure than motion palpation alone (k = 0.20 − 0.69) (Boline et al., 1988, 1993; Keating et al., 1990; Hubka, 1994; Hubka and Phelan, 1994; Nilsson, 1995). These authors conclude that palpation for cervical spine tenderness is a highly reliable examination tool and more promising than other pre-manipulative palpation methods.

It does appear that palpation for pain over both soft tissues and spinous processes is the only examination procedure to demonstrate any consistent inter-examiner reliability (Boline et al., 1988, 1993; McCombe et al., 1989; Keating et al., 1990). A recent intra-examiner reliability study on static palpation conducted by (O'Haire and Gibbons, 2000) studied the inter/intra-examiner reliability of 10 senior osteopathic students using static palpation on 10 asymptomatic subjects. The examiners had to palpate statically the posterior superior iliac spine (PSIS), sacral sulcus (SS) and the sacral inferior lateral angle (SILA), in the prone position. Sets of result cards were used for the examiners to record their findings. The results were consistent, in that the undergraduates, like previous studies but using post-graduates, showed poor inter-examiner reliability. The study failed to prove the reliability of static palpation of the (PSIS), (SS), and (SILA), as the kappa values did not exceed 0.08. However, intra-examiner agreement was greater than inter-examiner agreement, which is consistent with previous palpation reliability reports. McKenzie and Taylor (1997) also highlighted that intra-examiner analysis was supportive of the hypothesis that the same examiner could consistently palpate and find the same area of hypomobility. However, the reliability and validity of commonly used prone passive palpation methods have yet to be experimentally verified (Haas, 1992).

Therefore, it would seem reasonable to assume that more accurate anatomical and/or segmental localization protocols should be included in the methodological protocols of future reliability trials. Moreover, in communicating palpatory findings, is it necessary to locate and record accurately specific landmark identification? For clinical findings to be useful they have to be reasonably accurate if they are to be used in clinical trials (Breen, 1992). This assumes a certain degree of segmental specificity and accuracy that implies that spinal manipulation is precisely targeted at exact spinal segments (Haas et al., 1993). Furthermore, this also suggests that palpatory procedures must be equally as exact which may present an unattainable standard for determining reliability (Haas et al., 1995b). The precept of segmental specificity has yet to be clinically verified (Haas and Panzer, 1995).

The evidence regarding the objectivity of palpation does suggest some measure of inaccuracy in these techniques, which sheds some doubt on whether this is clinically a realistic assumption. The questions then arise:

- How critical is the accuracy or preciseness of segmental identification between examiners?
- What level of accuracy will be tolerated by therapeutic intervention in a clinical trial?

Poor agreement between experienced palpators has been demonstrated when comparing spinous process identification from the sitting to the prone posture (Byfield and Humphreys, 1992). The results of this study favoured bony landmark identification in the prone position using known anatomical reference points such as the pelvic crest. It has also been shown that greater error is associated with deeper and less clearly defined structures (Simmonds and Kumar, 1993; O' Haire and Gibbons, 2000).

Considering the fact that most motion palpation reliability studies to date have been performed in the sitting posture and that the reliability and validity of prone palpation techniques have yet to be experimentally verified (Haas, 1992), this indicates that improved methodological design incorporating these findings may improve overall clinical outcomes.

Therefore, accurate and repeatable segmental identification could be considered a prerequisite for critical evaluation of motion palpation (Byfield and Mathiasen, 1991; Byfield and Humphreys, 1992; Byfield et al., 1992; Haas and Panzer, 1995).

Perhaps it is less important that clinicians identify the correct segmental level provided they can agree on the same one. This may imply that what one observer calls L3 and another as L2 could in fact be the same targeted segment. Breen (1992) reiterated that the ability to locate an anatomical structure is by no means secure. If acceptably high levels of reliability could be achieved with a plus or minus one segment error being tolerated, this would have important consequences for validation procedures, since the naming of the segmental level is not essential, especially when targeting spinal manipulative therapy. Moreover, the level of agreement between myofascial trigger points and intersegmental fixations was recently shown to be 79% for exact level and one segment above and below (Vernon et al., 1990). This segmental specificity standard continues to challenge the rigorous and clinical expectations set down by the chiropractic profession.

Summary

Palpation of the spine and extremities is still a very common procedure in clinical back pain management. Moreover, despite its widespread use, the reliability and validity of palpation procedures is considered to be somewhat dubious, guesswork at best, in light of the overwhelming lack of experimental confirmation as a stand alone diagnostic tool (Troyanovich et al., 1998).

Furthermore, no validated 'gold standard' or reference measure against which to assess and/or confirm palpation accuracy has been experimentally determined (Mootz et al., 1989; Nansel et al., 1989; Haas et al., 1995b) and this needs to be studied further (van der Wurff, 2000b). It has been stated that the lack of a validated standard is not considered a limitation in palpation reliability trials, but rather a hindrance in concurrent validity trials (Keating, 1992). Moveover, it has also been reported that, in the absence of an established standard measure of spinal joint restriction (criterion validity), it is mandatory that high levels of inter-examiner reliability be demonstrated prior to defining any clinical relevance (Nansel et al., 1989). To date this has not been demonstrated, as inter-examiner consistency is considered no better than a chance occurrence. Apart from one study which utilized a questionable external standard (manipulation) to investigate the construct validity of end-play palpation (Haas et al., 1995b), there have been no other validity studies concerning motion palpation accuracy. Notwithstanding, the face (content) validity of motion palpation is currently strong but few conclusions regarding the clinical utility of motion palpation procedures can be made at this time (Keating, 1988c). Validity assessment is therefore considered to be a more crucial factor particularly as reliability is not a sufficient condition for validity (Wright and Feinstein, 1992).

In addition, no strong quantitative data exist regarding what constitutes an intersegmental joint restriction (fixation) even though a plethora of qualitative criteria are well described and documented. This may have contributed to poor inter-examiner communication and clinical interpretation, which may constitute another important confounding factor influencing palpation objectivity. Common terms such as joint fixation have only been addressed in and between examiner reliability with inconclusive results. Moreover, a general lack of motion palpation skill standardization combined with varying teaching methodologies may have also contributed to the disappointing results regarding palpation diagnosis when attempting to compare the results of various studies. Proposing to isolate one diagnostic strategy experimentally may have misrepresented a typical clinical encounter and underestimated the true value of practitioner experience.

Therefore, it would be prudent to initiate the possibility of developing a prototype system or external reference standard (in vitro) against which to investigate directly the accuracy of palpation skills.

Most inter-examiner motion palpation reliability studies have demonstrated marginal concordance at best (Keating, 1989a, 1990). This should not be seen as a complete lack of palpatory reliability, as reasonably good intra-examiner (test-retest) reproducibility has been reported in some studies (Love and Brodeur, 1987; Panzer, 1992; McKenzie and Taylor 1997). For example, investigating more standardized sacroiliac joint (SI) palpation testing procedures (Gillet, 1960; Grice, 1980; Kirkaldy-Willis, 1988; Bernard and Cassidy, 1991) has resulted in both good intra- and respectable inter-examiner reliability

(Carmichael, 1987; Herzog et al., 1989). These results may have been enhanced by the fact that the posterior superior iliac spine (PSIS), used to identify SI joint location, is a highly accessible anatomical landmark (Byfield et al., 1992).

Furthermore, high specificity (ability to identify non-fixated normal joint mobility) was reported for these standard well-described sacroiliac motion palpation tests in a healthy population of chiropractic students (Wiles, 1980). These results were not duplicated in symptomatic subjects (low back pain), however, a high degree of palpation sensitivity (ability to determine a fixated joint/manipulable lesion) was reported (Brunarski, 1982).

The differences found thus far in most studies investigating concordance have been attributed to differences in practitioner palpation techniques (Wiles, 1980; Love and Brodeur, 1987; Jull et al., 1988; Mootz et al., 1989; Faye and Wiles, 1992; McKenzie and Taylor, 1997; O'Haire and Gibbons, 2000). This is not surprising considering that this diagnostic assessment method is dependent upon such complex variables as practitioner skill, specific technique, educational background and experience (Humphreys, 1996). However, Binkley et al. (1995) suggest there may not be a direct relationship between examiners' experience and inter-examiner reliability.

This may be confounded by the fact that there is not as yet a well documented standardized, valid or reliable set of palpatory indicators to identify spinal joint dysfunction against which palpation findings can be actually matched (reference criteria) (Mootz et al., 1989). Highly variable manual palpation techniques coupled with a lack of a professional standardized format of this 'art form' has, in part, contributed to these conflicting results. In order to address this issue, some authors proclaim that a shift away from documenting existing palpation techniques to validating a standardized set of reliable indicators of segmental dysfunction would partially eliminate some of the variability associated with palpation findings (Mootz et al., 1989). Others lean towards a more comprehensive qualitative educational process, which is mentor driven and student centred (Love and Brodeur, 1987). In contrast, it has been suggested that specific motion palpation techniques be identified and refined as a representative subset of examination techniques used in future studies as a gold standard (Faye and Wiles, 1992). Furthermore, other researchers propose that a balance between both a quantitative and qualitative approach be explored to direct future efforts and research including standardizing palpatory techniques, established palpation thresholds and identifying palpation methods which possess the most applicable characteristics to meet clinical objectives (Panzer, 1992; Humphreys, 1996). These authors tend to support a balanced view with a slightly greater emphasis towards the educational perspective. This should include agreement and professional consensus regarding clear, concise definitions of palpation terminology, methods and clinical objectives.

EDUCATIONAL CONSIDERATIONS

A recent opinion has called for the removal of motion palpation from the educational curriculum altogether (Troyanovich et al., 1998). The logic behind this argument is based upon the concept that if motion palpation is investigational, doubtful or inappropriate as a diagnostic tool then it should not be taught in educational institutions. However, if this reasoning stems from the lack of demonstrable reliability and validity of motion palpation, then it must be remembered that inter-examiner agreement is notoriously difficult to prove (Sackett, 1980). Furthermore, it should be noted that other medical disciplines have experienced similar difficulty in seemingly easily reproducible procedures, such as the assessment of airway obstruction (Mior et al., 1985). Therefore, the very fact that motion palpation has not been proved effective does not by definition mean that it is ineffective (Liebenson and Chapman, 1999). Moreover, as Pringle (1999) correctly suggests, lobbying for the removal of motion palpation from educational programs is illogical when studies such as that of Haas (1991a) have concluded that there are insufficient numbers of studies to draw any firm conclusions. The same author further concludes by suggesting that the root of the error associated with motion palpation stems from poor use of motor learning principles when teaching motion palpation.

From an educational perspective, very little is known concerning how students learn the complex psychomotor skills needed to perform motion palpation and spinal manipulative techniques (Humphreys, 1996). This process is both a complex and difficult task (Byfield, 1996).

Knowledge of results and internal proprioceptive feedback may be critical variables in the successful performance of various psychomotor skills (Winstein, 1991; Good, 1993). In terms of reinforcement, considerable uncertainty exists about which approach or strategy is optimal in practical situations (Watts, 1990). It appears that optimal results are achieved through continuous reinforcement in the initial learning stages to more infrequent and sporadic feedback as learning advances and skills are attained (Watts, 1990). Furthermore, teaching and learning complex psychomotor skills such as palpation diagnosis is an integration of specified skills, knowledge and clinical relevance (Humphreys, 1996).

With respect to psychomotor skills learning, knowledge of results or feedback on performance has been shown to enhance skill retention if provided in a random fashion with respect to learning manipulating techniques (Good, 1993). In fact, such variables as rate of learning and level of skill attained are directly related to knowledge of performance (Keating et al., 1993). Furthermore, it has been postulated that the nature of the type and quality of feedback is an important factor in acquiring complex manual skills (Lee et al., 1990). Moreover, the nervous system is designed in such a way that newly acquired skills are enhanced by appropriate feedback protocols (McCarthy, 1996).

Humphreys (1996) advocated the introduction of quantifying progress using in an educational setting for example, mechanical models, videos and in depth performance criteria to provide accurate feedback and reinforce skill attention. He reported that excessive feedback can inhibit skill retention, that if provided on a more timely intermittent basis it could enhance a student's learning experience.

Therefore, more traditional teaching methods which focus on visual demonstration and mass practice combined with delayed qualitative feedback may represent confounding variables during psychomotor skills learning (Keating et al., 1993; Byfield, 1996). Feedback at this level is essentially subjective showing significant variability (Watson and Burnett, 1990). Notwithstanding, there is some speculation that one important factor contributing to such high inter-examiner variability may be directly related to current teaching methods. These methods may lack objective quantitative measurement of skills acquisition during the initializing phase (Love and Brodeur, 1987; Mootz et al., 1989; Harvey and Byfield, 1991; Keating et al., 1993; Byfield, 1996). Introducing clinically relevant examples (clinical frame-working), formulating step by step performance criteria and establishing valid and reliable feedback systems to measure skill acquisition has been proposed to enhance the learning experience (Lee et al., 1990; Keating et al., 1993; Simmonds et al., 1995; Humphreys 1996).

Therefore, it has been postulated that a standardized process and improved assessment protocols for associated psychomotor skills may be enhanced by employing mechanical models equipped with calibrated quantitative feedback systems (Haas and Panzer, 1995).

A number of studies have generated quantitative information regarding the forces and amplitudes involved in graded small amplitude passive movements of the spine similar to those used to perform Maitland graded mobilizations (Evans, 1986; Grieve and Shirley, 1987; Watson and Burnett, 1990; Lee and Evans, 1992; Keating et al., 1993; Simmonds et al., 1995). More consistent and accurate performance was noted immediately following experimental procedures and skills were still intact during follow up testing conducted at a later date (Lee et al., 1990; Keating et al., 1993). Watson and Burnett (1990) designed a mechanical device that was capable of measuring various grades of mobilization. Their results demonstrated considerable inter-therapist variability in the depth of all four Maitland mobilization grades (Watson and Burnett, 1990).

These results were echoed in a more recent study investigating both applied forces and the accuracy of therapists using a mechanical model (Simmonds et al., 1995). The results of this study showed that, in addition to high inter-therapist variability, there was a general underestimation of the amount of applied force and an overestimation of motion perceived by the therapists. Forces in the range of 58 to 178 newtons (N) were recorded across the Maitland mobilization grading system and individual therapists were regarded as the primary source of variability during force measurements (Simmonds et al., 1995).

Forces in the order of 200 N (45 lb) have been measured during application of graded oscillatory mobilization of the spine (Matyas and Bach, 1985). Even though they demonstrated a wide variation, the magnitude of these forces compared quantitatively with the preload forces measured during chiropractic manipulation of thoracic spine (Conway et al., 1993). It was determined that forces in the range of 400 N (90 lb) with a preload force of 145 N (33 lb) were required to cause joint cavitation during a manipulative thrust applied to this region of the spine (Conway et al., 1993). Depth measurements were not recorded, however, cavitation occurred just prior to peak force (Conway et al., 1993). In contrast, the magnitude of the thrust force recorded during prone posterior to anterior manipulation of the sacroiliac joints was in the range of 220 to 550 N (50–120 lb) (Hessel et al., 1990). It would appear that joint preload forces measured during similar posterior to anterior manipulative procedures are within an equivalent range for graded passive movements reported in the literature (Simmonds et al., 1995). These values may provide a benchmark for establishing a palpatory threshold to achieve during skill acquisition.

It does appear that there is significant variation between practitioners with regards to their perception of applied force and amplitude associated with both manipulative and mobilization procedures. Furthermore, there is significant potential for individual variation in the criteria incorporated by practitioners using palpatory diagnosis. This raises questions such as:

- What constitutes a segmental joint restriction or manipulable lesion?
- What would constitute a minimum palpatory force and depth threshold value when embarking on a standardization process for psychomotor skills acquisition?

Establishing valid and reliable benchmark values may strengthen psychomotor skills learning and initiate a more effective standardization process at the undergraduate level. Adding this objective dimension to already established cognitive and mental imagery teaching strategies may further enhance the learning experience and encourage the development of standardized palpatory criteria (Josefowitz et al., 1989; Stig et al., 1989).

To begin a standardization programme, one would need to determine the most commonly used motion palpation skills and procedures and determine which of those methods are most repeatable and useful from a diagnostic point of view. It may therefore be prudent for further replication on a wider geographical scale of the study compiled by Walker and Buchbinder (1997) that investigated the most commonly used methods of chiropractors in Victoria, Australia. Furthermore, the fact that the reliability and validity of commonly used passive prone palpation techniques and other static palpation methods have yet to be experimentally scrutinized may indicate that the full spectrum of available skills has yet to be fully explored (Haas, 1992). A general lack of communication when describing palpatory outcomes, as well as contradictory teaching methods, which are deficient in quantitative feedback, have been held responsible for the apparent disparity in most inter-examiner studies to date (Panzer, 1992). Practitioners may simply differ with respect to the amount of force and depth during palpation.

Variation in psychomotor skills and subsequent tactile perception across a wide range of palpation methods could explain the poor inter-observer reliability results reported in all regions of the spine. Although palpation type and protocols were explained and practised in these studies, it would be very difficult to assess in vivo consistency of palpatory depth, force applied against bony landmarks and ensure a valid recording (Byfield et al., 1995).

The subjects selected for this study (Byfield et al., 1995) had graduated from various chiropractic colleges and described various years of experience, some were practising part-time and others were not practising at all. Disparity in educational experience and exposure to various clinical definitions and terminology could influence palpatory skills, interpretation and inter-examiner outcome (Panzer, 1992). Recent attempts to clarify and redefine specific terms within the chiropractic profession, for example subluxation and fixation, have been well documented and clearly presented recently (Peterson and Bergmann, 1993; Gatterman, 1995). It is these specific definitions that should be included in future validity and reliability studies to establish clearly procedural and outcome parameters. This feature was consistently omitted in most methodological designs in previous trials, with the exception of Haas et al. (1995a, b) who defined their specific experimental palpation parameters. Most others used general terms which could be viewed as an important omission (Panzer, 1992). This could also be a plausible explanation for the recorded variation in the palpation parameters. Until more quantitative data can be obtained and validated, one cannot assess whether a subject is statistically more consistent than another.

Furthermore, a quantitative approach to palpation investigation may be able to address some of the points raised by Mior et al. (1990), regarding the role of clinical experience and specific teaching method and palpation reliability. It seems that experience did ensure some degree of palpation consistency, indicating that a certain level of psychomotor skill reproducibility and development is not affected over time when compared to the less experienced palpators as indicated by the experimental data to date. It may well be that variation in oscillatory pattern is more directly related to *specific chiropractic education than years of experience*. A future comparative study to determine any statistically significant differences and/or similarities between various levels of undergraduate skill and those that may exist between student and clinician may identify specific requirements with respect to undergraduate training methods.

The use of such an instrumented device to quantify specific chiropractic diagnostic palpation parameters has been documented (Byfield et al., 1994, 1995). Furthermore, palpation simulators have also been used to generate quantitative information with respect to/and limited to forces and amplitudes involved in graded small calibre passive movements of the spine (Maitland graded oscillations) (Evans, 1986; Grieve and Shirley, 1987; Evans et al., 1988; Watson and Burnett, 1990; Simmonds et al., 1995). In each case, the equipment demonstrated considerable inter-examiner variation in the measured parameters. Evans (1986) reported that the palpation simulator did show that a trained manipulative therapist performed more accurately than untrained subjects, suggesting that such systems could be used in the training of palpation skills. Similar findings with respect to experience were also demonstrated in the present study. It has been shown that providing quantitative feedback on performance significantly improves both accuracy and consistency of Maitland grade II mobilizing forces (Lee et al., 1990). This has meaningful implications with respect to the use of mechanical models at the educational level with respect to standardizing psychomotor skills including perception of forces and displacement associated with motion palpation and other palpation procedures (Byfield et al., 1995).

Mechanical devices may play a future role in the learning of palpation skills as both a teaching and an assessment tool (Byfield et al., 1995). There is a clear need to quantify specific palpation parameters as an integral component of the educational and standardization process. It is envisaged that the need for this process will take place at the undergraduate level by introducing a viable feedback system providing quantitative information regarding the acquisition and assessment of psychomotor aspects of motion palpation procedures (Humphreys, 1996). Even though discrepancies will always exist within any diagnostic system, students should have the opportunity to establish a baseline from which they may further develop their palpatory skills and overall appreciation of segmental dysfunction. Establishing a minimum/maximum threshold range with respect to palpation forces and depth may provide a reference point against which psychomotor skills can be more accurately assessed at the undergraduate level (Byfield et al., 1995). This work is continuing to progress and has been reported at a number of recent professional meetings.

The proposed threshold range should be based upon the values determined in previous studies

(Simmonds et al., 1995) and combined with further experimentation of the existing palpation apparatus. The upper limit should be formulated from known data regarding the forces required to cause joint cavitation during spinal manipulation of various regions of the spine (Hessell et al., 1990; Conway et al., 1993). Furthermore, having a numerical range to compare skills acquisition would provide a preliminary platform for quantitative standardization of the psychomotor skills associated with both motion palpation and spinal mobilization/manipulation. Quantifying these clinical perceptions of tissue and/or joint movement would move the manual professions away from such a heavy reliance upon qualitative descriptions of common clinical entities. This would provide an opportunity to redefine complex and confusing terms, such as subluxation, joint fixation and manipulable lesion, in clear kinematic designations which should help consolidate various interpretations presently in existence (Gatterman, 1995).

FINAL SUMMARY

Palpation still remains an integral part of a chiropractic clinical examination and many chiropractors continue to use it because it 'works for them' (Lucas, 2000). Reliable and valid measurements are essential components of research and clinical practice in the manipulative sciences (Campbell, 1987). Furthermore, reliability is regarded as a minimal requirement for both accurate and credible clinical outcomes (Wright and Feinstein, 1992). To date, the literature has reported that palpation and motion palpation methods for all regions of the spine are inconsistent and regarded as no better than a shot in the dark and as such may only contribute marginally to the decision making process. Experimental design, statistical analysis and interpretation of the results are still heavily debated and unresolved (Keating, 1989b; Carmichael, 1989; Haas and Nyiendo, 1990, 1991; Nansel et al., 1990; Haas, 1991d; Lantz, 1991). There are a number of very good reasons why it is essential that reliability be improved, most notably, justifying continued use of motion palpation, enhancing overall palpation accuracy in terms of therapeutic appropriateness and monitoring clinical changes over time (Haas and Panzer, 1995). Therefore, until sound objective testing is performed, the diagnostic value and utility of motion palpation will remain untenable. On the other hand, good inter-examiner concordance has been demonstrated for locating spinal and soft tissue tenderness in both the lumbar and cervical spines (Boline et al., 1993; Hubka and Phelan, 1994; Downey et al., 1999). Traditionally regarded as highly subjective, palpation for pain may be the most objective pre-manipulative indicator and outcome measure at this time. Furthermore, considering its widespread use, no attempts quantitatively to correlate palpation findings with the manipulable lesion in a controlled trial have been initiated. Future controlled trials investigating the efficacy of manipulative therapy should include spinal monitoring protocols that incorporate both pain location and motion analysis in combination as multiple test regimens.

Moreover, just because there is no reliability does not necessarily mean that the phenomenon does not exist. Nonetheless, if we cannot agree we cannot be accurate, especially when two examiners at any given time completely disagree with each other, which raises the question, are we simply more reliable than the research shows? It would appear that, despite lack of any conclusive empirical support, the face (content) validity of motion palpation procedures remains unblemished. This is further strengthened by the appearance of several recently published textbooks, review articles and other publications covering a wide range of palpation protocols, many of which have been cited in this chapter. This may represent attempts by educators, clinicians and researchers alike to standardize various motion palpation methods and experimental methodology which has been highlighted and referred to as a source of failure in early reliability studies. The construct validity of motion palpation has also received encouragement recently, following favourable short-term responsiveness reported in a study which analysed end-play methods before and after manipulation in the thoracic spine (Haas et el., 1995b). This signifies an important transgression from investigating examination tools in isolation that has dominated most palpation reliability/validity trials to date. These researchers attempted to investigate motion palpation within more clinically relevant boundaries reinforcing the concept of combined reliability.

The evidence clearly indicates that the specificity of motion palpation has yet to be experimentally established in vitro. The results of repeat trials using an articulated spinal model could indicate that motion palpation appears to be a specific rather than a sensitive method of spinal analysis. These conclusions should be viewed with caution, particularly in light of the fact the model failed to simulate a sense of realism for palpation procedures. Naturally, there were some who have questioned the purpose and contribution of such models

(Simmonds et al., 1995) and there were those who have fully supported this paradigm (Love and Brodeur, 1987; Panzer, 1992; Leach, 1994; Haas and Panzer, 1995).

Regardless of these differences of opinion, the introduction of models capable of quantifying palpation skills adds a measure of objectivity to the investigative process. At this stage it can only be concluded that, with respect to joint play methods, considerable variability exists between examiners with respect to their perception of palpation forces and depth of deformation. The results of this study warrants further exploration regarding psychomotor skill acquisition and assessment. Additional development of such models may play a key role in standardizing and assessing palpation skills during the initializing phase at the undergraduate level. Clearly defined palpation terminology and operational criteria that reflect concepts of joint analysis, which are consistent with known kinematic and intrinsic soft tissue characteristics should drive this review. Formulating the most efficient motion palpation that reflects the most dominant kinematic movement as compared to testing all ranges regardless, may eliminate some confusion and redundancy. Utilizing various palpating positions (sitting, supine and prone) would permit analysis of all aspects of the active, passive and accessory movements prior to therapeutic selection.

As part of the rigorous standardization process, a review of the segmental specificity assumption should be included in this audit. With very few exceptions, reliability has been evaluated within the confines of specific segment by segment analysis. Since this has not been shown to be valid, examiners may only have to agree on a specific region in order to establish acceptable concordance and reflect procedural accuracy (Haas et al., 1993). Increasing the palpation zone may increase the overall reliability. This point was demonstrated during palpation trials using the articulated spinal device when the zone of accuracy for correct fixation identification was extended to one segment above or below the targeted motion segment. Naturally, it would be easier to substantiate agreement over a wider range of segments than segment by segment. A future study utilizing this regional approach to fixation analysis combined with DVF technology could shed more light on palpation validity.

Standards of practice and clinical guidelines are becoming a normal part of responsible professional conduct and demanded by both public and private concerns. Standardization of our most commonly used diagnostic tools is foremost in that growth.

This chapter has demonstrated that palpation procedures are a very complex learned set of psychomotor skills that are influenced by a number of various clinical interactions. Understanding these processes may be supported through the development of reliable quantification systems that can measure clinical events and enhance overall patient care.

REFERENCES

Acker, P'., Thiel, H., Kirkaldy-Willis, W.H. (1990) Low back pain: pathogenesis, diagnosis and management. *Am J Chiro Med.* **3**, 19–24.

Alley, R.J. (1983) The clinical value of motion palpation as a diagnostic tool: a review. *J Can Chiro Assoc.* **27**, 97–100.

American Chiropractic Association (ACA) Council on Technic (1988) Chiropractic terminology: a report. *J Am Chiro Assoc.* **25**(10), 46.

Banks, S., Willis. J.C. (1988) The validity of manual diagnosis. *Spinal Manipulation.* **9** (3), 1–3.

Beal, M.C. (1953) Motion sense. *J Am Osteo Assoc.* **53**, 151–153.

Belski, S.E. (1988) Letter to the editor. *J Manipulative Physiol Ther.* **11**, 53.

Bergmann, T.F., Peterson, D.H., Lawrence, D.J. (1993) *Chiropractic Technique.* Churchill Livingstone, London.

Bergmann, T.F., Peterson, D.H. (1995) Joint assessment principles and procedures. In: *Proceedings of Technique Tune-up: From Palpation to Cavitation* CMCC/OCA Conference, Toronto.

Bergstrom, E., Courtis, G.W. (1986) An inter- and intra-examiner reliability study of motion palpation of the lumbar spine in lateral flexion in the seated position. *Eur J Chiro.* **34**, 121–141.

Bernard, T.N., Cassidy, J.D. (1991) The sacroiliac syndrome: pathophysiology, diagnosis, and management. In: *The Adult Spine* (Frymoyer, J.W. ed.) pp. 2107–2130. Raven Press, New York.

Binkley, J., Stratford, P., Gill, C. (1995) Interrater reliability of lumbar accessory motion mobility testing. *Physical Therapy.* **75**, 786–792.

Bogduk, N., Twomey, L.T. (1987) Nerves of the lumbar spine. In: *Clinical Anatomy of the Lumbar Spine* (Bogduk, N., Twomey, L.T. eds) pp. 92–102. Churchill Livingstone, London.

Boline, P.D., Keating, J.C., Brist, J., Denver, D. (1988) Interexaminer reliability of palpatory evaluation of the lumbar spine. *Am J Chiro Med.* **1**(1), 5–11.

Boline, D.B., Haas, M., Meyer, J.J., Kassak, K., Nelson, C., Keating, J.C. (1993) Interexaminer reliability of eight evaluative dimensions of lumbar segmental abnormality: part II. *J Manipulative Physiol Ther.* **16**, 363–374.

Breen, A. (1977) Chiropractic in Britain. *Ann Swiss Chiropractors' Assoc.* **VI**, 46–53.

Breen, A. (1992) The reliability of palpation and other diagnostic methods. *J Manipulative Physiol Ther.* **15**, 54–57.

Brunarski, D.J. (1982) Chiropractic biomechanical evaluations: validity in myofascial low back pain. *J Manipulative Physiol Ther.* **5**, 155–161.

Burton, A.K., Edwards, V., Sykes, D.A. (1990) 'Invisible' skin marking for testing palpatory reliability. *J Man Med.* **5**, 1–3.

Byfield, D., Mathiasen, J. (1991) A preliminary study investigating the accuracy of bony landmark identification in the lumbar spine. *Eur J Chiro.* **39**, 105–109.

Byfield, D., Humphreys, K. (1992) Intra- and inter-examiner reliability of bony landmark identification in the lumbar spine. *Eur J Chiro.* **40**, 13–17.

Byfield, D.C., Mathiasen, J., Sangren, C. (1992) The reliability of osseous landmark palpation in the lumbar spine and pelvis. *Eur J Chiro.* **40**, 83–88.

Byfield, D., Burnett, M., Ellis, R., McCarthy, P., Mealing, D. (1994) A feasibility study of a spinal model design to investigate the threshold and reliability of passive joint play palpation. *J Manipulative Physiol Ther.* **17**, 273–274.

Byfield, D. (1994) Letter to the editor. *Eur J Chiro.* **42**, 55–56.

Byfield, D., Burnett, M., Mealing, D., Ellis, R., McCarthy, P. (1995) Quantifying simulated joint play palpation using an instrumental device. *Eur J Chiro.* **43**, 47–53.

Byfield, D. (ed.) (1996) Introduction. In: *Chiropractic Manipulative Skills.* pp. 1–8. Butterworth-Heinemann, Oxford.

Campbell, S.K. (1987) On the importance of being earnest about measurement, or, how can we be sure that what we know is true? *Phys Ther.* **67**, 1831–1833.

Carmichael, J. (1987) Inter- and intra-reliability of palpation for sacroiliac joint dysfunction. *J Manipulative Physiol Ther.* **10**, 164–171.

Carmichael, J. (1989) Letter to the editor. *J Manipulative Physiol Ther.* **12**, 156–158.

Cassidy, J.D., Theil, H.W., Kirkaldy-Willis, W.H. (1993) Side posture manipulation for lumbar intervertebral disc herniation. *J Manipulative Physiol Ther.* **16**, 96–103.

Cibulka, M.T., Delitto, A., Koldenhoff, R.M. (1988) Changes in innominate tilt after manipulation of the sacroiliac joints in patients with low back pain: an experimental study. *Phys Ther.* **68**, 1359–1363.

Conway, P.J.W., Herzog, W., Zhang, Y., Hasler, E.M., Ladly, K. (1993) Forces required to cause cavitation during spinal manipulation of the thoracic spine. *Clin Biomechanics.* **8**, 210–214.

Cyriax, J. (ed.) (1975) The diagnosis of soft tissue lesions. In: *Textbook of Orthopaedic Medicine,* 6th edn. pp. 61–98. Bailliere Tindall, London.

DeBoer, K.F., Harmon, R., Tuttle, C.D., Wallace, H. (1985) Reliability study of detection of somatic dysfunction in the cervical spine. *J. Manipulative Physiol Ther.* **8**, 9–16.

Dishman, R.W. (1988) Static and dynamic components of the chiropractic subluxation complex: a literature review. *J Manipulative Physiol Ther.* **11**, 98–107.

Downey, B.J., Taylor, N.F., Niere, K.R. (1999) Manipulative physiotherapists can reliably palpate nominated lumbar spinal levels. *Man Ther.* **4**, 151–156.

Evans, D.H. (1986) The reliability of assessment parameters: accuracy and palpation technique. In: *Modern Manual Therapy of the Vertebral Column* (Grieve, G.P., ed). pp. 498–502. Churchill-Livingstone, Edinburgh.

Evans, D.H., Trott, P.H., Pugatschew, A., Baghurst, P. (1988) Manual palpation of resistance to movement. Parts 1 & 2 A study of the skills of manipulative therapists. In: *Proceedings of the International Federation of Orthopaedic Manipulative Therapists Congress.* Cambridge.

Faye, L.J., Wiles, M.R. (1992) Manual examination of the spine. In: *Principles and Practice of Chiropractic* (Haldeman, S., ed.). pp. 301–318. Appleton & Lange, San Mateo, California.

Feinstein, R.A. (1985) *Clinical Epidemiology: The architecture of Clinical Research.* W.B. Saunders, Philadelphia.

Fligg, D.B. (1984) The art of motion palpation. *J Can Chiro Assoc.* **28**, 331–334.

French, S.D., Green S., Forbes, A. (2000) Reliability of chiropractic methods commonly used to detect manipulable lesions in patients with chronic low back pain. *J Manip Physiol Ther.* **23**, 231–238.

Galley, P.M., Forster, A.L. (1987) Basic principles of mechanics. In: *Human Movement: An Introductory Test for Physiotherapy* (Streiner, D.L., Norman, G.R., eds). pp. 79–96. Oxford University Press, Oxford.

Gatterman, M.I. (ed.) (1995) What's in a word? In: *Foundations of Chiropractic Subluxation.* pp. 5–17. Mosby, Toronto.

Gillet, H. (1960) Vertebral fixations, an introduction to movement palpation. *Ann Swiss Chiro Assoc.* **I**, 30.

Gillet, H., Leikens, M. (1969) A further study of spinal fixations. *Ann Swiss Chiro Assoc.* **IV**, 41.

Gitelman, R. (1980) A chiropractic approach to biomechanical disorders of the lumbar spine and pelvis. In: *Modern Developments in the Principles and Practice of Chiropractic* (Haldman, S. ed.). pp. 297–330. Appleton-Century-Crofts, New York.

Gonnella, C., Paris, S., Kutner, S. (1982) Reliability in evaluating passive intervertebral motion. *Phys Ther.* **62**, 436–444.

Good, C.J. (1993) Aspects of learning issues relevant to the chiropractic adjustment. *J Chiro Ed.* September, pp. 59–68.

Greenman, P.E. (ed.) (1989a) Structural diagnosis and manipulative medicine. In: *Principles of Manual Medicine.* pp.1–12. Williams & Wilkins, London.

Greenman, P.E. (ed.) (1989b) Principles of structural diagnosis. In: *Principles of Manual Medicine.* pp.13–30. Williams & Wilkins, London.

Grice, A. (1979) Radiographic, biomechanical and clinical factors in lumbar lateral flexion. *J Manipulative Physiol Ther.* **2**, 26–34.

Grice, A. (1980) A biomechanical approach to cervical and dorsal adjusting. In: *Modern Developments in the Principles and Practice of Chiropractic* (Haldeman, S., ed.). pp. 331–339. Appleton-Century-Crofts, New York.

Grieve, G.P., Shirley, A.W. (1987) The measurement of pressures used in simulated passive accessory oscillatory mobilization techniques. In: *Proceedings of World Congress, Confederation for Physical Therapy*, Sydney.

Haas, M., Nyiendo, J. (1990) Letter to the editor. *J Manipulative Physiol Ther.* **13**, 346.

Haas, M., Nyiendo, J., Peterson, C. et al. (1990) Inter-rater reliability of roentgenological evaluation of the lumbar spine in lateral bending. *J Manipulative Physiol Ther.* **13**, 179–189.

Haas, M. (1991a) The reliability of reliability studies. *J Manipulative Physiol Ther.* **14**, 199–208.

Haas, M. (1991b) Statistical methodology for reliability studies. *J Manipulative Physiol Ther.* **14**, 119–132.

Haas, M. (1991c) Interexaminer reliability for multiple diagnostic test regimens. *J Manipulative Physiol Ther.* **14**, 95–103.

Haas, M. (1991d) Letter to the editor. *J Manipulative Physiol Ther.* **14**, 331–333.

Haas, M., Nyiendo, J. (1991) Letter to the editor. *J Manipulative Physiol Ther.* **14**, 158–159.

Haas, M. (1992) Module summaries from consensus conference: module 3 summary: motion palpation of the lumbar spine. *Chiro Tech.* **4**, 38–40.

Haas, M., Peterson, D., Hoyer, D., Ross, G. (1993) The reliability of muscle testing response to a provocative vertebral challenge. *Chiro Tech.* **5**, 95–100.

Haas, M., Panzer, D.M. (1995) Palpatory diagnosis of subluxation. In: *Foundation of Chiropractic Subluxation* (Gatterman, M., ed.). pp. 56–67. Mosby, Toronto.

Haas, M., Raphael, R., Panzer, D., Peterson, D. (1995a) Reliability of manual end-play palpation of the thoracic spine. *Chiro Tech.* **7**, 120–124.

Haas, M., Panzer, D., Peterson, D., Raphael, R. (1995b) Short-term responsiveness of manual thoracic end-play assessment to spinal manipulation: a randomized controlled trial of construct validity. *J Manipulative Physiol Ther.* **18**, 582–589.

Harvey, D., Byfield, D. (1991) Preliminary studies with a mechanical model for the evaluation of spinal motion palpation. *Clin Biomechanics.* **6**, 79–82.

Hawk, C., Phongphua, C., Bleecker, J., Lopez, D., Rubley, T. (1999) Preliminary study of the reliability of assessment procedures for indications for chiropractic adjustments of the lumbar spine. *J Manipulative and Physiol Ther.* **22**, 382–389.

Hersboek, L., Lebouef-Yde, C. (2000) Are chiropractic tests for the lumbo-pelvic spine reliable and valid? A systematic critical literature review. *J Manipulative Physiol Ther.* **23**, 258–275.

Herzog, W., Read, L.J., Conway, P.J.W., Shaw, L.D., McEwen, M.C. (1989) Reliability of motion palpation procedures to detect sacroiliac joint fixations. *J Manipulative Physiol Ther.* **12**, 86–92.

Hessell, B.W., Herzog, W., Conway, P.J.W., McEwan, M.C. (1990) Experimental measurement of the force exerted during spinal manipulation using the Thompson Technique. *J Manipulative Physiol Ther.* **13**, 448–453.

Hubka, M.J. (1994) Palpation for spinal tenderness: a reliable and accurate method for identifying the target of spinal manipulation. *Chiro Tech.* **6**, 5–8.

Hubka, M.J., Phelan, S.P. (1994) Inter-examiner reliability of palpation for cervical spine tenderness. *J Manipulation Physiol Ther.* **17**, 591–595.

Humphreys, K. (1996) Educational aspects of the teaching and learning of skills. In: *Chiropractic Manipulative Skills* (Byfield, D., ed.). pp. 9–21. Butterworth-Heinemann, Oxford.

Jansen, R.D., Nansel, D.D. (1988) Diagnostic illusions: the reliability of random chance. *J Manipulative Physiol Ther.* **11**, 355–361.

Jensen, K.J., Gemmell, H., Thiel, H. (1993) Motion palpation accuracy using a mechanical spinal model. *Euro J Chiro.* **41**, 67–73.

Johnston, W.L. (1975) The role of static and motion palpation in structural diagnosis. *J Am Osteo Assoc.* **75**, 421–424.

Johnston, W.L. (1982) Passive gross motion testing examiner agreement on selected subjects. *J Am Osteo Assoc.* **81**, 309–313.

Josefowitz, N., Stermac, L., Grice, A., Fligg, B., Moss, J., Szaraz, Z. (1986) Cognitive imagery in learning chiropractic skills: the role of imagery. *J Can Chiro Assoc.* **30**, 195–199.

Jull, G., Bogduk, N., Marsland, A. (1988) The accuracy of manual diagnosis for cervical zygaphophysial joint pain diagnosis. *Med J Aust.* **148**, 233–236.

Kaltenborn, F., Lindahl, O. (1969) Reproducerbatheten vid rorelseuder solininh av enskilda kotor. *Lakartidningen.* **66**(10), 962–965.

Keating, J.C. (1988a) Several strategies for evaluating the objectivity of measurements in clinical research and practice. *J Can Chiro Assoc.* **32**, 133–138.

Keating, J.C. (1988b) Letter to the editor. *J Manipulative Physiol Ther.* **11**, 53–56.

Keating, J.C. (1988c) Letter to the editor. *J Manipulative Physiol Ther.* **11**, 443–444.

Keating, J.C. (1989a) Inter-examiner reliability of motion palpation of the lumbar spine: review of the literature. *Am J Chiro Med.* **2**, 107–110.

Keating, J.C. (1989b) Letter to the editor. *J Manipulative Physiol Ther.* **12**, 155–156.

Keating, J.C., Bergmann, T.F., Jacobs, G.E., Finer, B.A., Larson, K. (1990) Interexaminer reliability of eight evaluative dimensions of lumbar segmental abnormality. *J Manipulative Physiol Ther.* **13**, 463–470.

Keating, J., Matyas, T.A., Bach, T.M. (1993) The effect of training on physical therapist's ability to apply specified forces of palpation. *Phys Ther.* **73**, 45–53.

Keating, J.C. (ed.) (1992) Some interferential statistics for measurement evaluation. In: *Toward a Philosophy of the Science of Chiropractic: A Primer for Clinicians.* pp.157–184.

Stockton Foundation for Chiropractic Research, Stockton, California.

Kessler, R.M. (1983) Assessment of musculoskeletal disorders. In: *Management of Common Musculoskeletal Disorders* (Kessler, R.M., Hertling, D., eds). pp. 75–104. Harper & Row, London.

Kirkaldy-Willis, W.H., Cassidy, J.D. (1985) Spinal manipulation in the treatment of low back pain. *Can Fam Phys.* **31**, 535–540.

Kirkaldy-Willis, W.H. (ed.) (1988) The site and nature of the lesion. In: *Managing Low Back Pain.* pp.133–154. Churchill-Livingstone, London.

Kondracki, M. (1996) Some biomechanical considerations in manipulative skills training. In: *Chiropractic Manipulative Skills* (Byfield, D., ed.). pp. 22–31. Butterworth-Heinemann, Oxford.

Koran, L.M. (1975b) The reliability of clinical methods, data and judgements (second of two parts). *New Eng J Med.* **293**, 695–701.

Lantz, C.A. (1991) Letter to the editor. *J Manipulative Physiol Ther.* **14**, 329–330.

Leach, R.A. (ed.) (1994) Soft outcome measures of dysfunction. In: *The Chiropractic Theories Principles and Clinical Application* 3rd edn. pp. 55–71. Williams & Wilkins, London.

Leboeuf, C., Gardner. V., Carter, A.L., Scott. T.A. (1989) Chiropractic examination procedures: a reliability and consistency study. *J Aust Chir Assoc.* **19**, 101–104.

Lee, M., Moseley, A., Refshauge, K. (1990) Effect of feedback on learning a vertebral joint mobilization skill. *Phys Ther.* **70**, 45–50.

Lee, R., Evans, J. (1992) Load-displacement-time characteristics of the spine under posteroanterior mobilization. *Aust Physio.* **38**(2), 115–123.

Liebenson, C.S. (1992) Pathogenesis of chronic pain. *J Manipulative Physiol Ther.* **15**, 299–308.

Liebenson, C., Chapman, S. (1999) Motion palpation: It's time to accept the evidence. Letter to the editor. *J Manipulative Physiol Ther.* **22**, 631–633.

Lindh, M. (1989) Biomechanics of the lumbar spine. In: *Basic Biomechanics of the Musculoskeletal System*, 2nd edn (Nordin, M., Frankel, V., eds). pp. 183–207. Lea & Febiger, London.

Love, R., Brodeur, R. (1987) Inter- and intra-examiner reliability of motion palpation for thoracolumbar spine. *J Manipulative Physiol Ther.* **10**, 1–4.

Loebl, W.Y. (1967) Measurement of spinal posture and range of spinal movement. *Ann Phys Med.* **9**, 103–110.

Lovell, F.W., Rothstein, J.M., Personius, W.J. (1989) Reliability of clinical measurements of lumbar lordosis taken with a flexible rule. *Phys Ther.* **69**, 96–102.

Lucas, N.P. (2000) Motion palpation: It's time to accept the evidence. Letter to the editor. *J Manipulative Physiol Ther.* **23**, 60–61.

Lysell, E. (1969) Motion in the cervical spine. *Acta Ortho Scand.* **23** (Suppl), 1–61.

Maclure, M., Willet, W.C. (1987) Misinterpretation and misuse of the kappa statistic. *Am J Epidem.* **126**, 161–169.

Magee, D.J. (ed.) (1987) Principles and concepts. In: *Orthopaedic Physical Assessment.* pp. 1–20. W.B. Saunders Company, London.

Mann, M., Glasheen-Wray, M., Nyberg, R. (1984) Therapist agreement for palpation and observation of iliac crest heights. *Phys Ther.* **64**, 334–338.

Matyas, T.A., Bach, T.M. (1985) The reliability of selected techniques in linical arthrometrics. *Aust. J Physio.* **31**, 175–199.

Mayer, T.G., Tencer, T.F., Kristofersson, S., Monney, V. (1984) Use of non invasive techniques for quantification of spinal range of motion in normal subjects and chronic low back dysfunction patients. *Spine.* **9**, 558–595.

McCarthy, P.W. (1996) The physiology of skill performance. In: *Chiropractic Manipulative Skills* (Byfield, D., ed.). pp. 32–43. Butterworth-Heinemann, Oxford.

McCombe, P.F., Fracs, J.C.T., Fairbank, M.D., Cockesole, B.C., Pynsent, P.B. (1989) Reproducibility of physical signs in low back bain. *Spine.* **14**, 908–918.

McKenzie, A., Taylor, N. (1997) Can physiotherapists locate lumbar spinal levels by palpation? *Physiotherapy.* **83**, 235–239.

Mennell, J.M. (ed.) (1960) Movement, dysfunction, manipulation, spinal movement. In: *Back Pain: Diagnosis and Treatment using Manipulative Technique.* pp.14–28. Little, Brown and Company, Toronto.

Mennell, J.M. (ed.) (1964) Preamble. In: *Joint Pain: Diagnosis and Treatment using Manipulative Techniques.* pp.1–11. Little Brown & Company, Boston.

Mennell, J.M. (1990) Another critical look at the diagnosis 'joint dysfunction' in the synovial joints of the cervical spine. *J Manipulative Physiol Ther.* **13**, 7–12.

Mennell, J.M. (1991) The manipulable lesion: joint play, joint dysfunction and joint manipulation. In: *Functional Soft Tissue Examination and Treatment by Manual Methods* (Hammer, W., ed.). pp. 191–196. Aspen Publishers, Gaithersburg.

Mior, S.A., King, R.S., McGregor, M., Bernard, M. (1984) Intra and interexaminer reliability of motion palpation of the cervical spine. *J Can Chiro Asoc.* **29**, 195–198.

Mior, S.A., McGregor, M., Schut, A.B. (1990) The role of experience in clinical accuracy. *J Manipulative Physiol Ther.* **13**, 68–71.

Moll, J.M.H., Wright, V. (1971) Normal range of spinal mobility: an objective clinical study. *Ann Rheum Dis.* **30**, 381–385.

Mootz, R.D., Keating, J.C., Kontz, H.P., Milus, T.B., Jacobs, G.E. (1989) Intra- and inter-examiner reliability of passive motion palpation of the lumbar spine. *J Manipulative Physiol Ther.* **12**, 440–445.

Moroney, S.P., Schultz, A.B., Miller, J.A.A. (1988) Load-displacement properties of the lower cervical spine motion segments. *J Biomech.* **21**, 769–779.

Nansel, D.D., Jansen, R.D. (1988) Concordance between galvanic skin response and spinal palpation findings in pain-free males. *J Manipulative Physiol Ther.* **11**, 267–272.

Nansel, D.D., Peneff, A.L., Jansen, R.D., Cooperstein, R. (1989) Interexaminer concordance in detecting joint play asymmetries in the cervical spines of otherwise asymptomatic subjects. J Manipulative Physiol Ther. **12**, 428–433.

Nansel, D.D., Jansen, R.D., Peneff, A.L., Cooperstein, R. (1990) Letter to the editor. J Manipulative Physiol Ther. **13**, 346–349.

Nilsson, N. (1995) Measuring cervical muscle tenderness: a study of reliability. J Manipulative Physiol Ther. **18**, 88–90.

Norkin, C.C., Levangie, P.M. (eds) (1992) The vertebral column. In: Joint Structure and Function – A Comprehensive Analysis, 2nd edn. pp. 125–177. F.A. Davis Company, Philadelphia.

O'Haire, C., Gibbons, P. (2000) Inter-examiner and intra-examiner agreement for assessing sacroiliac anatomical landmarks using palpation and observation: pilot study. Manual Ther. **5**, 13–20.

Panjabi, M.M., Summers, D.J., Pelker, R.R. (1986) Three dimensional load displacement curves of the cervical spine. J Orth Res. **4**, 152–161.

Panjabi, M.M. (1992) The stabilizing system of the spine. Part 1. Function dysfunction, adaptation and enhancement. Part 2. Neutral zone and instability hypothesis. J Spinal Disorders. **5**, 383–397.

Panzer, D.M. (1992) The reliability of lumbar motion palpation. J Manipulative Physiol Ther. **15**, 518–524.

Paydar, D., Thiel, H., Gemmell, H. (1994) Intra- and inter-examiner reliability of certain pelvic palpatory procedures and the sitting flexion test for sacroiliac joint mobility and dysfunction. J Neur Musculoskeletal System. **2**, 65–69.

Peterson, D.H., Bergmann, T.F. (1993) Joint assessment principles and procedures. In: Chiropractic Technique (Bergmann, T.F., Peterson, D.H., Lawrence, D.J., eds). pp. 51–121. Churchill Livingstone, London.

Peterson, D.H. (1993) Principles of adjustive technique. In: Chiropractic Technique (Bergmann, T.F., Peterson, D.H., Lawrence, D.J., eds). pp. 123–196. Churchill Livingstone, London.

Pope, M.H., Wilder, D.G., Stokes, I.A.F., Frymoyer, J.W. (1977) Biomechanical testing as an aid to decision making in low back pain patients. Spine. **4**, 135–140.

Potter, R., Rothstein, J. (1985) Intertester reliability for selected tests of the sacroiliac joint. Phys Ther. **65**, 1671–1675.

Pringle, R.K. (1999) Motion palpation: It's time to accept the evidence. Letter to the editor. J Manipulative Physiol Ther. **22**, 181–182.

Rhudy, T.R., Sandefur, M.R., Burk, J.M. (1988) Interexaminer/intertechniques reliability in spinal subluxation assessment: a multifactorial approach. Am J Chiro Med. **1**, 111–114.

Russell, R. (1983) Diagnostic palpation of the spine: a review of procedures and assessment of their reliability. J Manipulative Physiol Ther. **6**, 181–183.

Sackett, D.L. (1980) Clinical disagreement: How often it occurs and why. Can Med Assoc J. **123**. 499–504.

Sandoz, R. (1976) Some physiological mechanisms and effects of spinal adjustments. Ann Swiss Chiro Assoc. **VI**, 91–142.

Schafer, R.C., Faye, L.J. (eds) (1989) The basic clinical approach in dynamic chiropractic. In: Motion Palpation and Chiropractic Technic – Principles of dynamic chiropractic. pp. 1–74. Motion Palpation Institute, Huntington Beach, California.

Simmonds, M.J., Kumar, S. (1993) Location of body structures by palpation – a reliability study. Int J Ind Ergonom. **11**, 145–151.

Simmonds, M.J., Kumar, S., Lechelt, E. (1995) Use of a spinal model to quantify the forces and motion that occur during therapist's tests of spinal motion. Phys Ther. **75**, 212–222.

Stig, L., Christensen, H.W., Byfield, D., Sasnow, M. (1989) Comparison of the effectiveness of physical practice and mental practice in the learning of chiropractic adjustive skills. Eur J Chiro. **37**, 70–76.

Stokes, I.A.F., Wilder, D.G., Frymoyer, J.W., Pope, M.H. (1981) Assessment of patients with low back pain by biplanar radiographic measurement of intervertebral motion. Spine. **6**, 233–240.

Stokes, I.A.F., Bevin, T.M., Lunn, R.A. (1987) Back surface curvature and measurement of lumbar spinal motion. Spine. **12**, 355–361.

Stokes, I.A. (1988) Mechanical function of the facet joints in the lumbar spine. Clin Biomechanics. **3**, 101–105.

Streiner, D.L., Norman, G.R. (eds) (1989) Reliability. In: Health Measurement Scales: A Practical Guide to Their Development and Use. pp. 79–96. Oxford University Press, Oxford.

Strender, L-E., Sjoblom, A., Sundell, K., Ludwig, R., Taube, A. (1997) Inter-examiner reliability in physical examination of patients with low back pain. Spine. **22**, 814–820.

Toussaint, R., Gawlik, C.S., Rehder, U., Ruther, W. (1999) Sacroiliac joint diagnostics in the Hamburg construction workers study. J. Manipulative Physiol Ther. **22**, 139–143.

Triano, J.J. (1990) The subluxation complex: outcome measure of chiropractic diagnosis and treatment. Chiro Tech. **2**, 114–117.

Troyanovich, S.J., Harrison, D.D., Harrison, D.E. (1998) Motion palpation: It's time to accept the evidence. J Manipulative Physiol Ther. **21**, 568–571.

Tuchin, P., Hart, C., Johnson, C. et al. (1996) Interexaminer reliability of chiropractic evaluation for cervical spine problems – a pilot study. Australasian Chiro Osteo. **5**, 23–29.

Van der Wurff, P., Hagmeijer, R.H.M., Meyne, W. (2000a) Clinical tests of the sacroiliac joint a systematic methodological review. Part 1. Reliability. Manual Ther. **5**, 30–36.

Van der Wurff, P., Hagmeijer, R.H.M., Meyne, W. (2000b) Clinical tests of the sacroiliac joint a systematic methodological review. Part 2. Validity. Manual Ther. **5**, 89–96.

Vernon, H., Cote, P., Beauchemin, D., Bonnoyer, B. (1990) A correlative study of myofascial tender points and joint fixations in the lumbar pelvic spine in low back pain. In: *Proceedings of the 1990 International Conference on Spinal Manipulation.* pp. 236–240. Foundation for Chiropractic Education and Research, Washington DC.

Walker, B.F. (1996) Spinal subluxation an overview of the literature. *Austalasian Chiro Osteo.* **5**, 12–22.

Walker, B.F., Buchbinder, R. (1997) Most commonly used methods of detecting spinal subluxation and the preferred term for its description: A survey of chiropractors in Victoria, Australia. *J Manipulative Physiol Ther.* **20**, 583–589.

Watson, M.J., Burnett, M. (1990) Equipment to evaluate the ability of physiotherapists to perform graded postero-anterior central vertebral pressure type passive movements of the spine by thumb pressure. *Physiotherapy.* **76**, 611–614.

Watts, N.T. (ed.) (1990) The events of learning and functions of teaching. In: *Textbook of Clinical Teaching.* pp. 24–27. Churchill Livingstone, London.

White, A.A., Panjabi, M. (eds) (1990) Kinematics of the spine. In: *Clinical Biomechanics of the Spine,* 2nd edn. pp. 61–86. J.B. Lippincott Company, Philadelphia.

Wiles, M.R. (1980) Reproducibility and inter examiner correlation of motion palpation findings of the sacroiliac joints. *J Can Chiro Assoc.* **24**, 59–69.

Winstein, C.J. (1991) Knowledge of results and motor learning – implications for physical therapy. *Phys Ther.* **71**, 140–149.

Wright, J.G., Feinstein, A.R. (1992) improving the reliability of orthopaedic measurements. *J Bone Surg (Br).* **74B**, 287–291.

Yamamota, I., Panjabi, M., Crisco, T., Oxland, T. (1989) Three dimensional movements of the whole lumbar spine and lumbosacral joint. *Spine.* **14**, 1256–1260.

FURTHER READING

Adams, A.H. (1990) Determining the usefulness of diagnostic procedures and tests. *Chiro Tech.* **2**, 90–93.

Allbrook, D. (1957) Movements of the lumbar spinal column. *J Bone Joint Surg.* **398**, 339–345.

Anderson, J.A.P., Sweetman, B.J. (1975) A combined flexirule/hydrogoniometer for the measurement of the lumbar spine and its sagittal movement. *Rheum Rehab.* **14**, 173–179.

Bartko, J.J., Carpenter, W.T. (1976) On the methods and theory of reliability. *J Nerv Ment Dis.* **163**(5), 307–317.

Bishop, R.G., Byfield, D., Bolton, J.E. (1991) A preliminary investigation into the relationship between lumbar sagittal mobility and pelvic mobility. *Eur J Chiro.* **39**, 3–11.

Blunt, K.L., Gatterman, M.I., Bereznick, D.E. (1995) Kinesiology; an essential approach toward understanding the chiropractor subluxation. In: *Foundations of Chiropractic Subluxation* (Gatterman, M.I., ed.). pp. 190–224. Mosby, Toronto.

Bolton, J.E. (1993) Methods of assessing low back pain and related psychological factors. *Eur J Chiro.* **41**, 31–38.

Breen, A., Allen, R., Morris, A. (1988) An image processing method for spine kinematics: preliminary studies. *Clin Biomechanics.* **3**, 5–10.

Breen, A., Allen, R., Morris, A. (1989) Spine kinematics: a digital videofluoroscopic technique. *J Biomed Eng.* **11**, 224–228.

Breen, A.C., Brydges, R., Kause, J., Allen, R. (1993) Quantitative analysis of lumbar spine intersegmental motion. *Phys Med Res.* **3**, 182–190.

Burton, A.K. (1986) Regional lumbar sagittal mobility: measurement by flexicurves. *Clin Biomechanics.* **1**, 20–26.

Burton, A.K., Tillotson, K.M. (1988) Reference values for normal regional lumbar sagittal mobility. *Clin Biomechanics.* **3**, 106–113.

Byfield, D.C., Harvey, D. (1991) Preliminary studies with mechanical model for the evaluation of spinal motion palpation. *Clin Biomechanics.* **6**, 79–82.

Cassidy, J.D., Potter, G.E. (1979) Motion examination of the lumbar spine. *J Manipulative Physiol Ther.* **2**, 151–158.

Cassidy, J.D., Kirkaldy-Willis, W.H., McGregor, M. (1985) Spinal manipulation for the treatment of chronic low back pain: an observational study. In: *Empirical Approaches to the Validation of Spinal Manipulation* (Buerger, A.A., Greenman, P.E., eds). pp. 123–128. Charles C. Thomas, Springfield IL.

Cohen, J. (1990) A coefficient of agreement for nominal scales. *Ed Psychol Measurement.* **20**, 37–46.

Deyo, R., Diehl, A.K. (1983) Measuring physical and psychosocial function in patients with low back pain. *Spine.* **8**, 635–642.

Deyo, R.A., McNiesh, L.M., Cone, R.O. (1985) Observer variability in the interpretation of lumbar spine radiographs. *Arth Rheum.* **28**(9), 1066–1070.

Deyo, R.A. (1988) Measuring the functional status of patients with low back pain. *Arch Phys Med Rehab.* **69**, 1044–1053.

Fitzgerald, G.K., Wynveen, K.J., Rhault, W., Rothschild, B. (1983) Objective assessment with establishment of normal values for lumbar spine range of motion. *Phys Ther.* **63**, 1776–1781.

Gatterman, M.I. (ed.) (1990) *Chiropractic Management of Spine Related Disorders.* Williams & Wilkins, London.

Gill, K., Kray, M.H., Johnson, G.B., Haugh, L.D., Pope, M.H. (1988) Repeatability of four clinical methods for the assessment of lumbar spinal mobility. *Spine.* **13**, 50–53.

Good, A.B. (1985) Spinal joint blocking. *J Manipulative Physio Ther.* **8**, 1–8.

Good, C.J., Eaton, S. (1994) Letter to the editor. *Eur J Chiro.* **42**, 56–57.

Greenman, P.E. (ed.) (1989a) Structural diagnosis and manipulative medicine. In: *Principles of Manual Medicine.* pp.1–12. Williams & Wilkins, London.

Gregerson, G.G., Lucas, D.B. (1967) An in-vivo study of the axial rotation of the human thoracolumbar spine. *J. Bone Joint Surg.* **49**(2), 247–262.

Griffen, A.B., Troup, J.D.G., Lloyd, D. (1984) Tests of lifting and handling capacity. *Ergonomics.* **27**, 305–320.

Gunzburg, R., Hutton, W., Fraser, R. (1991) Axial rotation of the lumbar spine and the effect of flexion. An in vitro and in vivo biomechanical study. *Spine.* **16**, 22–28.

Haley, S.M., Osberg, J.S. (1989) Kappa coefficient calculation using multiple ratings per subject: a special communication. *Phys Ther.* **69**, 90–94.

Herzog, W., Conway, P.J., Kawchuk, G.N., Zhang, Y., Hasler, E.M. (1993) Forces exerted during spinal manipulation therapy. *Spine.* **18**, 1206–1212.

Hindle, R.J., Pearcy, M.J., Cross, A.T., Miller, D.H.T. (1990) Three dimensional kinematics of the human back. *Clin Biomechanics.* **5**, 218–228.

Hubka, M.J. (1990) Another critical look at the subluxation hypothesis. *Chiro Tech.* **2**, 27–29.

Humphreys, K., Breen, A., Saxton, D. (1990) Incremental lumbar spine motion in the coronal plane: an observer variation study using digital videofluoroscopy. *Eur J Chiro.* **38**, 56–62.

Isreal, M. (1959) A quantitative method of estimating flexion and extension of the spine: a preliminary report. *Military Med.* **124**, 86–92.

Johnston, W.L. (1976) Interexaminer reliability in palpation. *J Am Osteo Assoc.* **76**, 286–287.

Jull, G., Bullock, M. (1987a) A motion profile of the lumbar spine in an ageing population assessed by manual examination. *Physiother Pract.* **3**, 70–81.

Jull, G., Bullock, M. (1987b) The influence of segmental level and direction of movement on age changes in lumbar motion as assessed by manual examination. *Physiother Pract.* **3**, 107–116.

Kappler, R.E. (1980) A comparison of structural examination findings obtained by experienced physician examiners and student examiners on hospital patients. *J Am Osteo Assoc.* **79**, 468–471.

Kawchuk, G.N., Herzog, W., Hasler, E.M. (1992) Forces generated during spinal manipulative therapy of the cervical spine: a pilot study. *J Manipulative Physiol Ther.* **15**, 275–278.

Koran, L.M. (1975a) The reliability of clinical methods, data and judgements (first of two parts). *New Eng J Med.* **253**, 642–646.

Kraemer, H.C. (1988) Assessment of 2 x 2 associations: generalization of signal-detection methodology. *Am Stat.* **42**, 37–49.

Liebenson, C., Phillips, R.B. (1989) The reliability of range of motion measurements for the lumbar spine flexion: a review. *Chiro Tech.* **1**, 69–78.

McConnell, D.G., Beal, M.C., Dinnar, U. et al. (1980) Low agreement of findings in neuromusculoskeletal examinations by a group of osteopathic physicians using their procedures. *J Am Osteo Assoc.* **79**, 441–450.

Mellin, G. (1986) Measurement of thoracolumbar posture and mobility with a myrin inclinometer. *Spine.* **11**, 759–762.

Mellin, G. (1989) Comparison between tape measurements of forward and lateral flexion of the spine. *Clin Biomechanics.* **4**, 121–123.

Mellin, G. (1990) Decreased joint and spinal mobility associated with low back pain in young adults. *J Spinal Disorders.* **3**, 238–243.

Norman, G.R., Streiner, D.C. (eds) (1986) Describing data. In: *PDQ Statistics.* pp.19–25. B.C. Decker Inc., Toronto.

Nunn, N.R. (1991) A study to investigate the reliability of detecting single and multiple motion restrictions in the lumbar spine using a mechanical model. Bsc. Project. Anglo-European College of Chiropractic, Bournemouth (D. Byfield, Supervisor).

Occipintie, E., Colombini, D., Menoi, O., Grieco, A. (1985) Alteration of the spine in the working population. 2: definite values for mobility of the vertebral column. *Medical Lav.* **76**, 509–515.

Pearcy, M.J., Tibrewal, S.B. (1982) Movement of the lumbar spine measured by three dimensional x-ray analysis. *J Biomed Eng.* **4**, 107–111.

Pearcy, M., Portek, I., Shepard, J. (1984) Three dimensional x-ray analysis of normal movement in the lumbar spine. *Spine.* **9**, 294–297.

Pearcy, M.J., Tibrewal, S.B. (1984) Axial rotation and lateral bending in the normal movement in the lumbar spine measured by 3-D radiography. *Spine.* **9**, 582–587.

Pearcy, M.J. (1985) Stereography of lumbar spine motion. *Acta Ortho Scand.* **56** (Suppl 212).

Pearcy, M., Portek, I., Shepard, J. (1985) The effect of low back pain on lumbar spinal movements measured by 3-D x-ray analysis. *Spine.* **10**, 150–153.

Pearcy, M.J. (1986) Measurement of back and spinal mobility. *Clin Biomechanics.* **1**, 44–51.

Pearcy, M.J., Gill, J.M., Hindle, R.J., Johnson, R.J., Johnson, G.R. (1987) Measurement of human back movements in three dimensions by opto electronic devices. *Clin Biomechanics.* **2**, 199–204.

Pearcy, M. (1989) Biomechanics of the spine. *Current Ortho.* **3**, 96–100.

Pearcy, M.J., Hindle, R.J. (1989) New method for the non invasive measurement of human back movements. *Clin Biomechanics.* **4**, 73–79.

Portek, I., Pearcy M.J., Reader, G.P., Mowat, A.G. (1983) Correlation between radiographic and clinical measurements of lumbar spine movement. *Brit J Rheum.* **22**, 197–205.

Rahlmann, J.F. (1987) Mechanisms of intervertebral joint fixation: a literature review. *J Manipulative Physiol Ther.* **10**, 177–187.

Rose, M.J. (1991) The statistical analysis of the intra-observer repeatability of four clinical measurement techniques. *Physiotherapy.* **77**, 89–91.

Rosner, B. (1986) *Fundamentals of Biostatistics,* 2nd edn. PWS Publisher, Boston.

Salisbury, P.J., Porter, R.W. (1987) Measurement of lumbar mobility a comparison of methods. *Spine.* **12**, 190–193.

Seigel, S., Castellan, M.J. (1988) *Non-Parametric Statistics for the Behavioural Sciences*, 2nd edn. McGraw-Hill, International Editions.

Soeken, K.L., Prescott, P.A. (1986) Issues in the use of kappa to estimate reliability. *Med Care.* **24**, 733–741.

Stokes, I.A.F., Medicott, P.A., Wilder, D.G. (1980) Measurement of movement in painful intervertebral joints. *Med Bio Eng Comput.* **18**, 694–700.

Stokes, I.A.F., Bevin, T.M., Lunn, R.A. (1987) Back surface curvature and measurement of lumbar spinal motion. *Spine.* **12**, 355–361.

Stokes, I.A. (1988) Mechanical function of the facet joints in the lumbar spine. *Clin Biomechanics.* **3**, 101–105.

Streiner, D.L., Norman, G.R. (eds) (1989) Reliability. In: *Health Measurement Scales: A Practical Guide to Their Development and Use.* pp. 79–96. Oxford University Press, Oxford.

Tanz, S.S. (1953) Motion of the lumbar spine. A roentgenologic study. *Am J Roentgen.* **69**, 399–412.

Taylor, J., Twomey, L. (1980) Sagittal and horizontal plane movement of the lumbar vertebral column in cadavers and the living. *Rheumat Rehab.* **19**, 223–231.

Thiel, H. (1994a) Reliability and validity of motion palpation procedures assessed on a mechanical spinal model. *J Manipulative Physiol Ther.* **17**, 290.

Thiel, H. (1994b) Letter to the editor. *Eur J Chiro.* **42**, 57–58.

Troup, J.D.G., Hood, C.A., Chapman, A.E. (1968) Measurements of the sagittal mobility of the lumbar spine and hips. *Ann Phys Med.* **9**, 308–321.

Troup, J.D.G., Forman, J.K., Baxter, C.E., Brown, D. (1987) The perception of back pain and the role of psychophysical tests of lifting capacity. *Spine.* **12**, 645–657.

Vernon, H. (1991) Chiropractic: a model of incorporating the illness behaviour model in the management of low back pain patients. *J Manipulative Physiol Ther.* **14**, 379–389.

Vernon, H. (1996) Pain and disability questionnaires in chiropractic rehabilitation. In: *Rehabilitation of the Spine: A Practitioner's Manual* (Liebensen, C., ed.). pp. 57–71. Williams & Wilkins, Baltimore.

Waddell, G.I., Main, C.J.M., Morris, E.W. et al. (1982) Normality and reliability in the clinical assessment of backache. *Brit Med J.* **284**, 1519–1523.

Waddell, G. (1987) A new clinical model for the treatment of low back pain. *Spine.* **12**, 632–636.

White, A.A., Panjabi, M.M. (1978) The basic kinematics of the human spine. A review of past and current knowledge. *Spine.* **3**, 12–20.

Zachman, Z.J., Bolles, S., Bergmann, T.F., Traina, A.D. (1989) Understanding the anterior thoracic adjustment: a concept of a sectional subluxation. *Chiro Tech.* Jan/Feb, 30–33.

2

Basic postural observation skills

David Byfield

By definition, posture is a state of muscular and skeletal balance that protects the supporting structures against injury or progressive deformity irrespective of its position (Bergmann et al., 1993). This description denotes the importance of posture with respect to efficient musculoskeletal function and its role in clinical practice and patient care. Moreover, analysis of posture is considered a common chiropractic examination procedure (Peterson and Bergmann, 1993), while from a scientific perspective, the reliability and validity of postural analysis as an examination procedure is equivocal at best. On the other hand, postural appreciation is considered to be an integral part of the assessment in a multidimensional diagnostic clinical index (Harrison et al., 1996; Vernon, 1999). Notwithstanding, a valid investigation of a patient's posture would require sophisticated equipment under controlled conditions, which is an unreasonable undertaking for a private practice environment. Gait analysis would be a good example of a complex and expensive analysis system. Simple methods, such as a vertical double plumbline, have been shown to be an effective clinical tool analysing posture before and after treatment intervention (Brunarski, 1982). Biological variation confounds any attempts to standardize posture analysis as a valid outcome measure of treatment effectiveness (Vernon, 1983).

Research has provided us with some objectivity with respect to postural assessment. Vernon (1995) and Vernon et al. (1999) found an association between faulty head posture (forward carriage) and a patient group suffering from chronic tension headaches. In addition, the validity of dynamic postural plumbline analysis has been investigated in its rela-

tionship to myofascial low back pain with some degree of consistency in identifying the impending symptomatic lesion (Brunarski, 1982). A four-quadrant weight scale designed to evaluate weight bearing in both the sagittal and frontal body planes was developed by the chiropractic profession but not studied in any great detail (Vernon and Grice, 1984). Vasilyeva and Lewit (1996) describe an entire system of diagnosing muscular dysfunction by postural inspection, but their systems have yet to be subjected to the rigours of a controlled clinical trial.

There has been an attempt to describe an ideally aligned static posture plus assessment protocols for interpreting static and dynamic modes for both the normal and abnormal states (Panzer et al., 1990; Sportelli and Tarola, 1992; Peterson and Bergmann, 1993). Apart from the purely observational exercise, these 'benchmarks' have not been subjected to appropriate scientific investigation nor tested as a valid outcome measure of treatment efficacy. The problem seems to lie in establishing a valid gold standard and correlating this benchmark to everyday life activities.

Static postural appreciation has limited association to daily life activities and correlates poorly with presenting symptoms. This may place some doubt upon its discriminant validity. Dynamic postural assessment, on the other hand, may provide additional functional patterns of movement but still lacks association with various activities of daily living and subsequently any real clinical relevance. Dynamic evaluation assesses movement in the sagittal and coronal planes relative to a reference plumbline in order to appreciate bilateral movement patterns and their possible clinical relationship. This may add another dimension to the clinical assessment and aid in establishing appropriate management plans for patient care.

Detecting normal symmetrical and asymmetrical patterns is an essential exercise during early examination skill training. This provides an excellent opportunity to integrate basic functional anatomy and clinical biomechanics. This chapter will outline the skills required to conduct a static and dynamic postural evaluation.

The chapter will be divided into three sections with and without plumbline evaluation.

1) *Static postural evaluation:*
   Posterior-anterior (P-A) view
   Anterior-posterior (A-P) view
   Lateral view
2) *Dynamic postural evaluation – standing:*
   Forward flexion
   Retroflexion
   Extension
   Lateral flexion
3) *Dynamic postural evaluation – sitting:*
   Forward flexion
   Lateral flexion

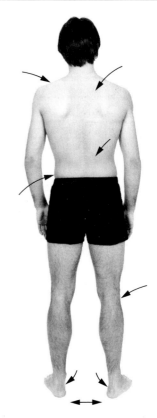

Fig. 2.1

1) STATIC POSTURAL EXAMINATION

Posterior-anterior view (P-A)

i)   Position the patient standing upright with the feet placed approximately hip distance apart facing forward. Observe the overall standing posture for general symmetry, any noticeable spinal curvatures or any obvious muscle imbalance (Figure 2.1). Note the posture of feet, taking note of the medial arch.

ii) Next have the patient laterally flex bilaterally to assess quality and quantity of movement (Figure 2.2a,b). Note the shape of the curve and the amount the hand reaches down the side of the leg (*).

iii) Ask the patient to bend forward and touch their toes to assess lumbopelvic flexion (Figure 2.3a). The movement should be symmetrical and midline with no deviations from the centre line (Figure 2.3b).

iv) Instruct the patient to extend backwards to assess the quality and quantity of movement (Figure 2.4a). Take note of the symmetry of the movement and the shape of the spine and the related soft tissues (Figure 2.4b).

v)   With the patient standing in front of a plumbline as a reference point, ensure that the feet are approximately hip distance apart. The plumbline should fall equidistant between the feet and bisect the gluteal crease, spinal midline and the head. This represents the postural gravity line and denotes relative symmetry in the coronal plane (Figure 2.5). General observation should include general skeletal symmetry, head position, ear lobe levels, shoulder levels, inferior scapular levels, pelvic crest levels, position of the popliteal creases, foot posture. Included in this observational exercise should be an appreciation of the overall muscular tone, spinal curvatures, any skin lesions and overall weight distribution.

vi) Observation begins systematically observing the position of the plumbline relative to various anatomical landmarks including the middle of the head, the external occipital protuberance down through the centre of the spinous processes of the cervicothoracic, midthoracic, thoracolumbar, lumbosacral, gluteal crease indicating postural symmetry and the presence of any spinal deviations from the postural gravity line (Figure 2.6).

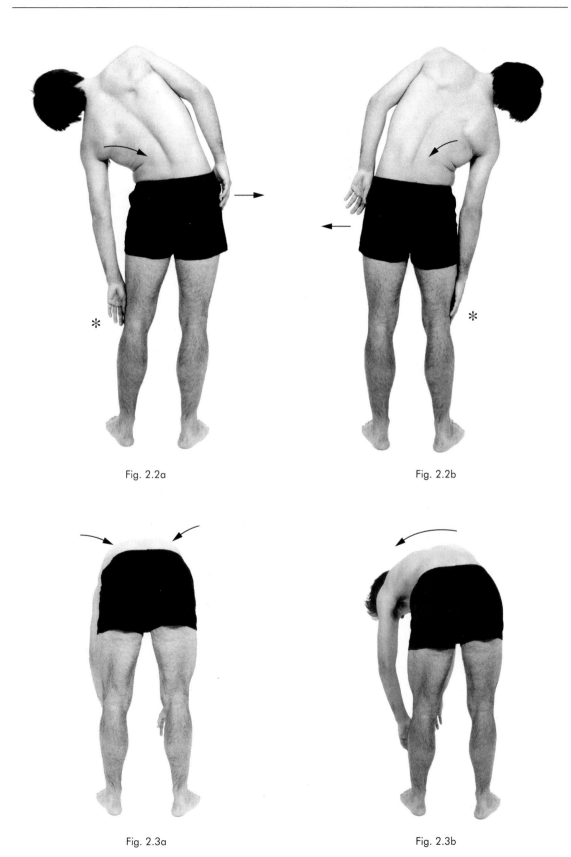

Fig. 2.2a

Fig. 2.2b

Fig. 2.3a

Fig. 2.3b

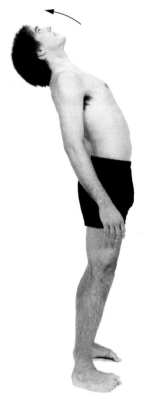

Fig. 2.4a

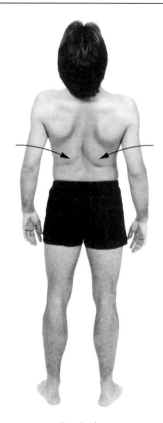

Fig. 2.4b

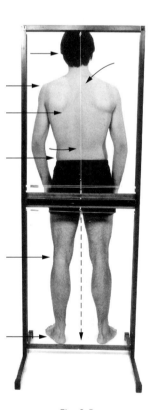

Fig. 2.5

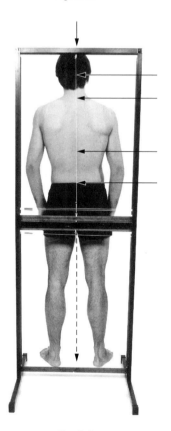

Fig. 2.6

Anterior-posterior view

i) Place the patient behind and facing the plumb-line with the line cutting through the feet placed approximately hip distance apart (Figure 2.7). Ideally, the plumbline should fall equally between the knees, pelvic region, umbilicus, sternum, chin, nose and forehead. Observe any asymmetrical deviation from the centre of the plumbline noting curvatures, muscle atrophy and general body alignment. Note the asymmetrical alignment in Figure 2.7.

ii) Once the P-A and A-P gravity lines have been established, the next step is to establish coronal plane symmetry by comparing various musculoskeletal landmarks and the anatomical postural gravity line including ear levels, shoulder levels, inferior scapula, pelvic crest posterior superior iliac spines (PSIS), gluteal fold, popliteal crease, Achilles tendon orientation and medial longitudinal arch formation (Figure 2.8).

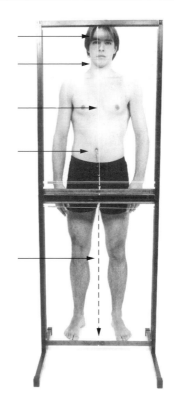

Fig. 2.7

Lateral view

i) Lateral gravity line appreciation begins by lining the plumbline just posterior to the styloid of the 5th metatarsal and slightly anterior to the ankle mortice joint. The line should then ideally fall just anterior to the centre of the knee joint, just posterior to the greater trochanter, through the middle of the pelvic crest, through the body of the 3rd lumbar vertebra, through the centre of the shoulder and through the external auditory meatus (Figure 2.9). This line provides a reasonably good appreciation of body weight distribution and possible regions of musculoskeletal stress.

2) DYNAMIC POSTURAL EXAMINATION – STANDING

Forward flexion – lateral view

i) With the patient standing lateral to the plumb-line, instruct the patient to bend forward slowly and touch their toes. During the initial movement observe flattening of the lumbar spine from the neutral (*) and the backward sway of the pelvis (Figure 2.10).

ii) Next observe rotation around the hip joints, forward tilt of the pelvis, relaxation of the hamstrings including the finger to floor dis-

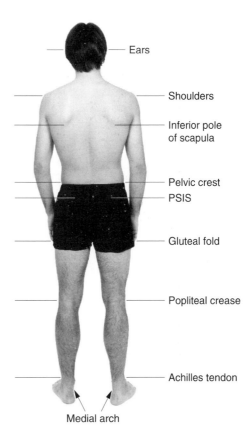

Ears

Shoulders

Inferior pole of scapula

Pelvic crest

PSIS

Gluteal fold

Popliteal crease

Achilles tendon

Medial arch

Fig. 2.8

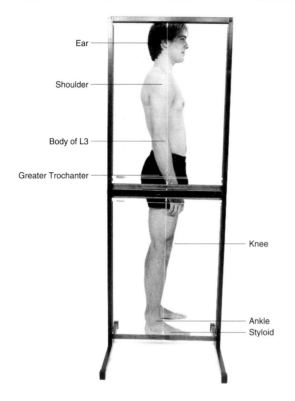

Ear

Shoulder

Body of L3

Greater Trochanter

Knee

Ankle
Styloid

Fig. 2.9

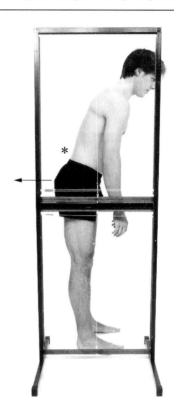

Fig. 2.10

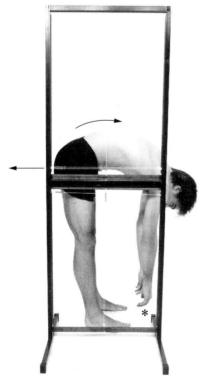

Fig. 2.11

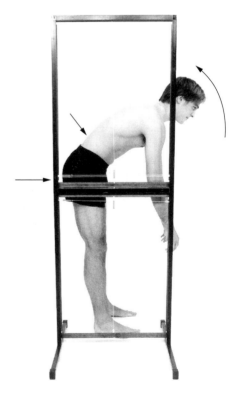

Fig. 2.12

tance (*) and overall movement pattern (Figure 2.11). This is known as lumbopelvic rhythm to balance the centre of gravity. Note approximate degree of overall flexion from the neutral posture.

iii) Instruct the patient to lift the trunk back up to the neutral from the fully flexed position (retroflexion) and observe the process in reverse noting any asymmetry of movement and the overall rhythm of movement and the re-establishment of the lumbar lordosis in order to maintain balance of the centre of gravity (Figure 2.12). Also observe the patient extending backwards from the neutral position on the plumbline as depicted in Figure 2.4a, b. Note general movement and overall symmetry.

iv) Note any deviation of the trunk from the midline during both forward and retroflexion to the neutral upright stance (Figure 2.13).

Backward extension – lateral view

i) From the neutral posture instruct the patient to bend backwards and extend the lumbar spine (see Figure 2.13). Observe pattern, rhythm and degree of movement.

Lateral flexion – posterior-anterior view

i) Place the patient in front of the plumbline in the neutral posture as in Figure 2.5. Instruct

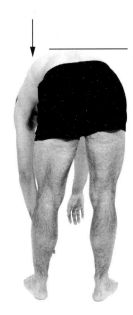

Fig. 2.13

the patient to bend laterally to the right following the hand down the side of the leg to its maximum point (Figure 2.14a). Note the degree of fingertip distance down the leg, C-curve in the lumbar spine (concavity on ipsilateral side of bending), amount of pelvic sway in each direction and the overall pattern of movement. The pelvic crests and PSIS should remain relatively level during this movement exercise (*). The plumbline should fall approximately through the ipsilateral gluteal region. Both left and right lateral flexion should be observed in order to ascertain the degree of bilaterally symmetrical movement (Figure 2.14b). This constitutes typical examination protocols. Note the differences between Figures 2.14a and 2.14b during lateral bending taking note of the amount of lateral sway bilaterally.

3) DYNAMIC POSTURAL EVALUATION – SITTING

Forward flexion

i) The patient should be sitting in a chair or stool. Note the upright sitting posture, taking note of the head position, shoulder alignment and the lumbar lordosis. Visualize an imaginary plumbline which should drop through the external auditory meatus and the centre of the shoulder (Figure 2.15).

ii) The patient is requested to bend forward noting the amount of flexion, the appearance of any spinal curvatures or lateral deviations compared with the standing examination (Figure 2.16). This exercise provides introductory differential diagnostic skills.

Lateral flexion

i) Note the patient sitting from behind, comparing any similarities or differences between the sitting and upright stances (Figure 2.17). Take note of any obvious spinal curvatures or deviation from an imaginary plumbline. Note the slight deviation of the head from the midline (*).

ii) With the patient sitting in an upright sitting posture ask them to bend sideways keeping their buttock firmly on the stool, first to the left (Figure 2.18a) and then to the right (Figure 2.18b). Note bilateral symmetry of

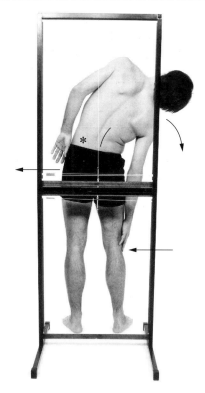

Fig. 2.14a

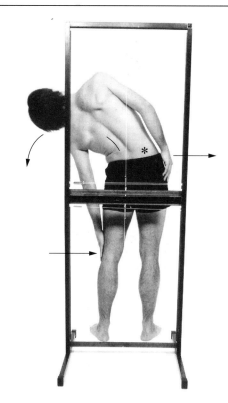

Fig. 2.14b

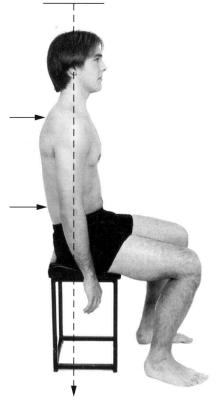

Fig. 2.15

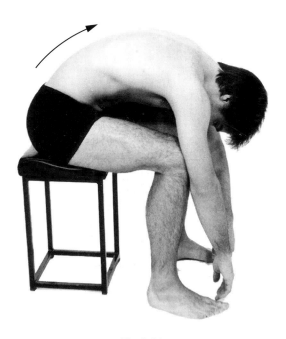

Fig. 2.16

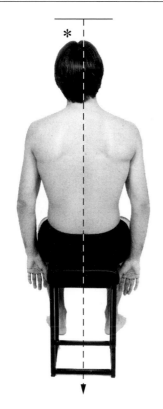

Fig. 2.17

movement, lumbar spinal C curve, amount of lateral flexion and any asymmetrical movements compared with the standing examination. These differences should be recorded accordingly.

SUMMARY

This chapter has presented some of the basic postural analysis skills commonly used in clinical practice. The presentation has also attempted to encapsulate foundational observational skills necessary during postural assessment to aid in the early development of clinical examination procedures.

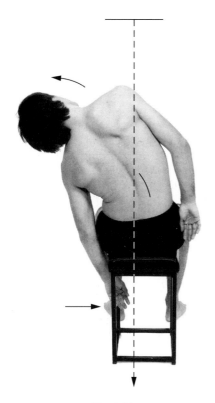

Fig. 2.18a

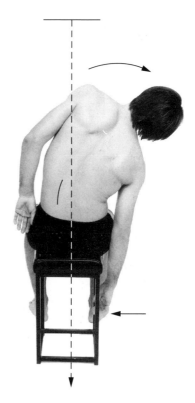

Fig. 2.18b

REFERENCES

Bergmann, T.F., Peterson, D.H., Lawrence, D.L. (eds) (1993) *Chiropractic Technique.* Churchill Livingstone, London.

Brunarski, D. (1982) Chiropractic biomechanical evaluations and validity in myofascial low back pain. *J Manipulative Physiol Ther.* **5**, 155–161.

Harrison, D.D., Janik, T.J., Harrison, G.R., Troyanovich, S., Harrison, D.E., Harrison, S.O. (1996) Chiropractic biophysics technique: a linear algebra approach to posture in chiropractic. *J Manipulative Physiol Ther.* **19**, 525–535.

Panzer, D.M., Fechtel, S.G., Gatterman, M.I. (1990) Postural complex. In: *Chiropractic Management of Spine Related Disorders* (Gatterman, M.I., ed.). pp. 256–284. Williams & Wilkins, London.

Peterson, D.H., Bergmann, T.F. (1993) Joint assessment principles and procedures. In: *Chiropractic Technique* (Bergmann, T.F., Peterson, D.H., Lawrence, D.L., eds). pp. 51–122. Churchill Livingstone, London.

Sportelli, L., Tarola, G.A. (1992) The history and physical examination. In: *Principles and Practice of Chiropractic,* 2nd edn. (Haldeman, S., ed.). pp. 261–300. Appleton & Lange, San Mateo, California.

Vasilyeva, L.F., Lewit, K. (1996) Diagnosis of muscular dysfunction by inspection. In: *Rehabilitation of the Spine: A Practitioner's Manual* (Liebenson, C., ed.). pp. 113–142. Williams & Wilkins, London.

Vernon, H. (1983) An assessment of the intra- and inter-reliability of the posturometer. *J Manipulative Physiol Ther.* **6**, 57–60.

Vernon, H. (1995) The effectiveness of chiropractic manipulation in the treatment of headache: an exploration in the literature. *J Manipulative Physiol Ther.* **18**, 611–617.

Vernon, H., Grice, A. (1984) The four quadrant weight scale: a technical and procedural review. *J Manipulative Physiol Ther.* **7**, 65–169.

Vernon, H., McDermaid, C.S., Hagino, C. (1999) Systematic review of randomized clinical trials of complementary/alternative therapies in the treatment of tension-type and cervicogenic headache. *Complément Ther Med.* **7**, 142–155.

FURTHER READING

Byfield, D. (1996) *Chiropractic Manipulative Skills.* Butterworth-Heinemann, Oxford.

Magee, D. (1987) *Orthopaedic Physical Assessment.* W.B. Saunders Company, London.

3

Basic lumbopelvic palpation and landmark identification skills

David Byfield

INTRODUCTION

Palpation of all the regions of the spine and pelvis is the most common examination procedure used by manipulative therapists to diagnose dysfunction of the vertebral motion segments. While clinicians have used both static and motion palpation procedures for over a century, the evidence based research studies have not been designed potentially to demonstrate the good reliability that practitioners report anecdotally. The lack of any convincing experimental consistency concerning palpation has been criticized by many as no better than chance occurrence. Furthermore, there have been very few studies concerning the clinical utility of static palpation procedures in relation to treatment outcomes. There are, however, some researchers who feel that the reliability of many of these palpatory skills may be enhanced when performed in combination with other assessment procedures as part of an overall examination profile. This provides more clinical 'reality' as clinicians rarely rely upon only one examination tool to formulate a clinical impression prior to any therapeutic intervention. This may certainly be the case, but in the meantime more trials are required to establish which assessment combinations provide valid and meaningful clinical information. It does appear that at present, static palpation procedures for pain and tenderness localization have demonstrated promising inter-observer concordance. This is encouraging but requires further clinical trials to establish whether or not soft tissue tenderness is a potential valid treatment outcome. In reality, it is the combination of assessment protocols, including the different palpation methods that one uses to glean information in as quick and efficient manner as possible.

Palpation of all the regions of the spine and pelvis with reference to specific anatomical landmarks and soft tissue configurations is a learned skill requiring many hours of practice and concentration. A strong basic anatomical knowledge must be established prior to embarking upon learning these psychomotor skill sets with any degree of proficiency. It has also been reported that visual and mental imagery may enhance complex psychomotor skill learning. Following appreciation of various structural markers, the next step is to introduce standard static palpation protocols to the dynamic qualities of the spinal and pelvic articulations. Lack of and/or aberrant articular movement has been identified as a fundamental prerequisite to spinal manipulative intervention. This analysis is underpinned by a descriptive theory outlining the active and passive range of motion of diarthroidal joints. It is also common practice to identify which particular holding elements (capsular and ligamentous) are challenged during each specific palpation procedure permitting the clinician to establish a reasonably accurate diagnosis of segmental diagnosis. The procedure should identify which aspect of the joint range of motion is impaired (active, passive, joint play, end play), the intersegmental level and potential pain generators.

This chapter will focus on two types of joint assessment: joint play and end feel (play). These are rudimentary joint analysis techniques and play an important role in establishing a clinical diagnosis in chiropractic practice. Joint play is described as the natural compliance of a joint in its neutral position (Peterson and Bergmann, 1993). End feel (play) is the assessment of the quality of the elastic barrier of the joint at the extent of the passive range prior to the paraphysiological space (Peterson and Bergmann, 1993). Joint play is performed in the neutral static posture while end play is performed at the end of the normal range of motion of a joint challenging the important support structures. This chapter will also focus on efficient ergonomics for the practitioner when learning and performing these basic palpatory skills for both the lumbar spine and pelvic regions. This chapter will also present a variety of soft tissue palpation techniques plus identification of a number of important anatomical landmarks in the lumbosacral region. Learning efficient postural skills during this process will provide the framework for more complex manipulative psychomotor skills implemented later during undergraduate education.

The chapter will present the following:

- Postural considerations – practitioner stance skills
- Soft tissue palpation and identification skills
- Anatomical landmark palpation and identification skills
- Joint play analysis skills of the lumbopelvic spine
- End play analysis skills of the lumbopelvic spine.

BASIC POSTURAL CONSIDERATION SKILLS – STANCE SKILLS

Efficient posture saves energy and protects the individual from developing overuse or repetitive strain symptoms. Learning to palpate is a complex skill including appropriate body stance and position capable of sustaining weight-bearing modes for several hours. With this in mind, good ergonomics implies learning the skills and knowledge associated with efficient posture and other work-related positions. This may reduce the risk of postural fatigue and commonly encountered practice-related back strain pain. Furthermore, these skills may develop awareness of body weight distribution in order to balance work postures. *This efficient body weight distribution is an important component of overall skill and performance to be adopted when learning palpation skills in all regions of the spine and pelvis described throughout this text.*

i) With the patient lying comfortably in the prone position, the practitioner should stand at 90 degrees to the table opposite the lumbopelvic region (Figure 3.1). The knees should be slightly flexed touching the lateral edge of the cushion. The table should support body weight in this position. The feet should be positioned approximately hip distance apart directly facing the table to ensure a stable base of support (*). The sternal notch should be aligned over the centre of the table to ensure body weight control.

ii) In order to project the body weight over the table to provide space for the hands to contact the intended landmark, flex the trunk slightly at the hips maintaining natural lordosis. The sternal notch (*) should be positioned directly over the lumbosacral spinal region (Figure 3.2). Note the position of the plumbline

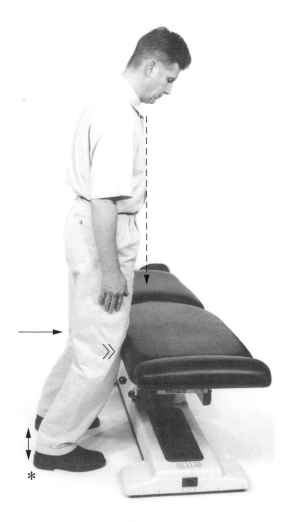

Fig. 3.1

(**). There should be spring in the legs to maintain balance and weight distribution. This is the ski *stance*, which is a basic posture and palpation position. This should be practised from both sides of the table. This is a basic palpation posture (Byfield, 1996).

iii) Once this basic ski stance has been accomplished, turn 45 degrees to the head of the table by pivoting on the metatarsal pads of the feet in one smooth motion to form the *fencer stance* (Figure 3.3). The fencer stance represents another important basic palpation and manipulative postural stance skill (Byfield, 1996). The weight is carried over the cephalad leg which is flexed (*) and the rear foot is plantar flexed (**) to push the weight forward over the table and spinal structures. This is an important movement during

manual skills development. Note the position of the sternal notch and palpating hands along with the slightly flexed trunk. The legs should remain flexible and the practitioner should lean slightly against the table to support overall body weight. Make sure that the back thigh is maintained perpendicular to the floor.

iv) Place the hands over the lumbosacral spine region making sure that the sternal notch and body weight distribution is aligned while still maintaining either the ski or fencer stances (Figure 3.4). Maintain plantar flexion of the rear foot at all times and spring over the front weight-bearing leg to ensure postural support (x). These skills should be practised from both sides of the table incorporating both stance options.

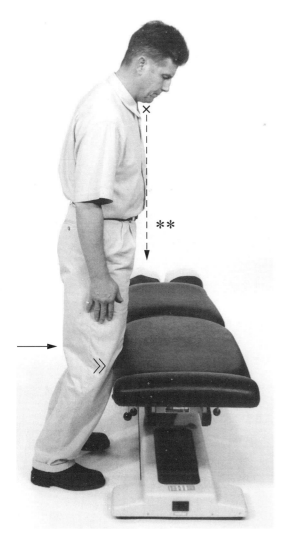

Fig. 3.2

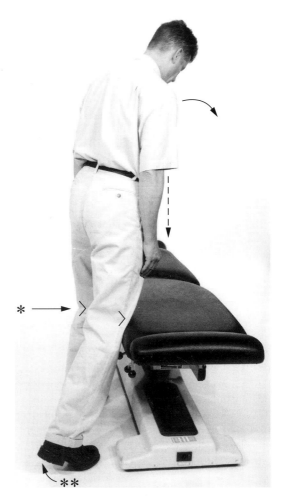

Fig. 3.3

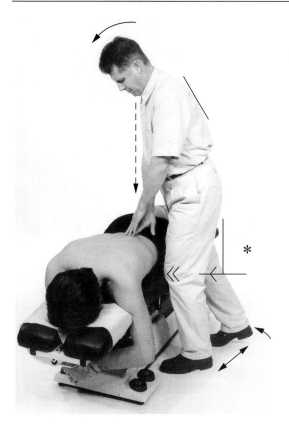

Fig. 3.4

ing temperature. Basic knowledge of the underlying anatomy will enhance palpation appreciation and recognition. The ability to acknowledge the normal tissue quality and texture is a preliminary step to differentiate various conditions and establish important decisions regarding a clinical impression and subsequent therapeutic pathways. Palpation for tissue tenderness has been shown to be very reliable between examiners in both the cervical and thoracic spines (Hubka, 1994). However, point tenderness has yet to be identified as a valid or reliable outcome measure in any randomized trial concerning the therapeutic efficacy of manual therapy. Needless to say, identifying localized tenderness is an essential component during a multidimensional diagnostic index of segmental dysfunction (Peterson and Bergmann, 1993). Regardless of its clinical utility, soft tissue palpation provides psychomotor skill training and provides information for clinical decisions.

The following will outline basic palpation skills and protocols for differentiating various tissue types and qualities. The emphasis will focus on a number of basic palpation skills necessary for early development and reinforcement.

Points to remember are to maintain:

  i) body weight against the table at optimal knee height
 ii) body symmetry/alignment
iii) sternal notch/chest cavity over the table and targeted joint
 iv) ensure that the feet stay approximately hip distance apart to maintain an adequate balance of the centre of gravity
  v) the thigh of the back leg should be perpendicular to the floor (Figure 3.4)(*).

SOFT TISSUE PALPATION AND BONY LANDMARK IDENTIFICATION

Examination of the skin and other soft tissue structures of the spine and pelvis are a fundamental assessment procedure. It also provides an opportunity for neophytes to begin a series of fundamental palpation procedures, including anatomical landmark location and soft tissue appreciation. It is important at the beginner level to distinguish between various tissue texture and quality includ-

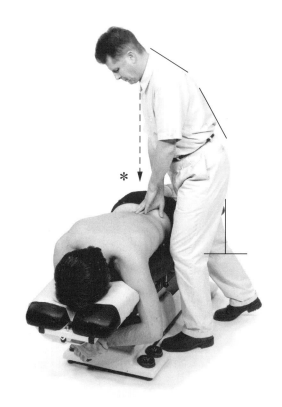

Fig. 3.5

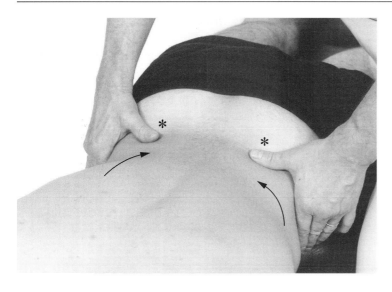

Fig. 3.6

Bony landmark location (spinous processes (SP), pelvic crest (PC), posterior superior iliac spine (PSIS), sacral tubercle (ST))

i)   Standing in either the ski stance (see Figure 3.2) or the fencer stance (see Figure 3.3) ensure that the sternal notch is located over the centre of the lumbosacral spine. Caution should be taken not to twist the spine, pelvis or shoulders during the stance at the table. Maintain symmetry, as this should position the palpating surface of the hands in an appropriate position (Figure 3.5). Maintain the sternal notch over the palpating fingers (*).

ii) Locate the most superior anterior edge of the pelvic (iliac) crest (PC) bilaterally by using the finger pads of the first and second digits, palpating from the front to the back, palpating the shape of the crest and including the bony contours of the iliac crest (Figure 3.6). Use the thumb of each hand to stabilize the palpating fingers during the exercise (*).

iii) As you continue, palpate the entire crest region and moving back and medially with the palpating fingers the innominate bone enlarges into a bony prominence, known as the PSIS, which is easily located with the thumb pads (*) (Figure 3.7). *Ensure that palpation is light but firm in order to appreciate the underlying osseous structures.*

iv) Probe the PSIS region. Replace the palpating fingers with the thumb pads to appreciate the contour and inferior ridge of the PSIS (Figure 3.8a). The PSIS varies in shape but has a prominent inferior edge (Figure 3.8b)(*). Ensure palpation is light and keep the sternal notch over the palpating fingers.

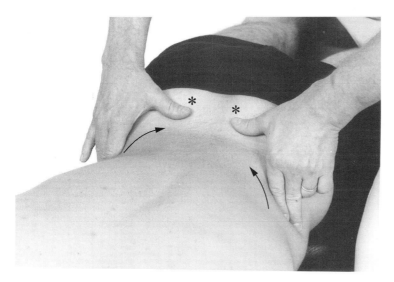

Fig. 3.7

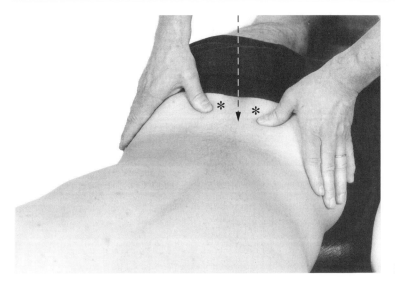

Fig. 3.8a

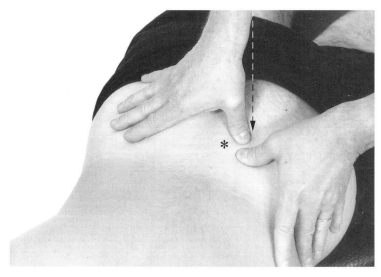

Fig. 3.8b

v) Following PSIS palpation move medially with the palpating thumb or fingers and locate the 2nd sacral tubercle (ST) located at the level of the inferior aspect of the PSIS (Figure 3.9). Continue to probe the 2nd sacral tubercle with the 1st and 2nd finger pads. This represents the sacral ridge and is considered the centre of axis of motion of the sacroiliac joint. Palpate the 1st sacral tubercle just cephalad to the 2nd. There should be a small indentation between the two tubercles.

vi) Palpate the SI joint line for symmetry bilaterally. The SI joint line is found just medial to the PSIS (Figure 3.10). Clinically this is a common area of pain or tenderness particularly associated with the long dorsal ligament which is located just inferior to the caudad portion of the PSIS.

vii) Continue to palpate caudally along the STs and then move laterally to the edge of the sacrum at the sacral angle (Figure 3.11a). As you continue to palpate around the lower lateral edge of the sacrum you will contact the sacral cornu and just inferior to this will be the sacrococcygeal joint (Figure 3.11b) (*).

viii) Standing in the fencer stance place both hands over the top of the iliac crest with both thumbs meeting in the midline. This should locate the inferior tip of the spinous process of L4 (Figure 3.12).

ix) With the caudad hand locate the interspinous space below L4 and the spinous process of L5. This will be more difficult to palpate due to the increased tissue mass in the region (Figure 3.13). *If there is difficulty palpating this region place a cushion under the*

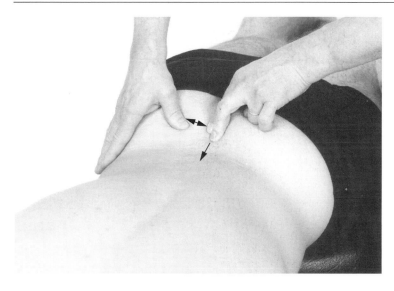

Fig. 3.9

patient's abdomen to raise the area and separate the spinous processes.

x) The L5 spinous process can also be located from the PSIS landmark and counting up from the 2nd ST (Figure 3.14).

xi) Begin to count the individual SPs in the lumbar spine beginning at L5 and working cephalad using the PSIS as a locating landmark (Figure 3.15).

xii) The palpation procedure should be done systematically by palpating the bony contour of each SP and the interspinous space that delineates each level with the palpating pad of each finger occupying an interspinous space (Figure 3.16). This exercise should continue to the thoracolumbar junction and above into the thoracic spine. The finger pads are most

adapted for this palpation exercise and the palpation should be light to appreciate the bony contours. Continue to count numerically until the thoracolumbar junction is reached at T12/L1 interspinous space.

xiii) This is the attachment for the 12th floating rib. Palpate laterally and bilaterally along the rib appreciating contour and overlying soft tissue (Figure 3.17).

Soft tissue palpation

i) From the fencer stance palpate the texture, contour and consistency of the immediate paraspinal soft tissues using the 1st and 2nd finger pads (Figure 3.18). Note the posture of the hands and fingers to the tissue surface (*).

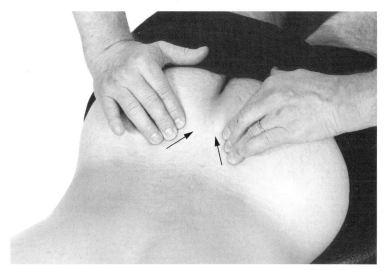

Fig. 3.10

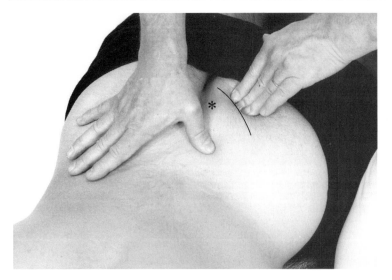

Fig. 3.11a

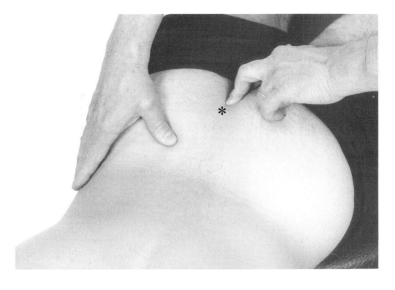

Fig. 3.11b

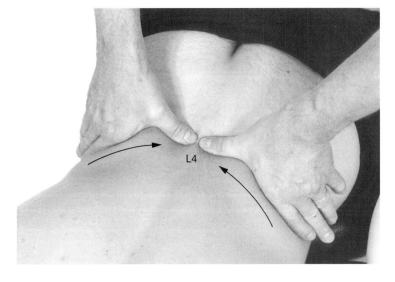

Fig. 3.12

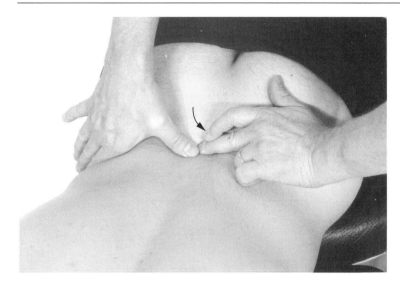

Fig. 3.13

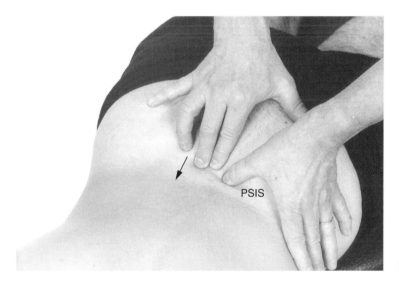

Fig. 3.14

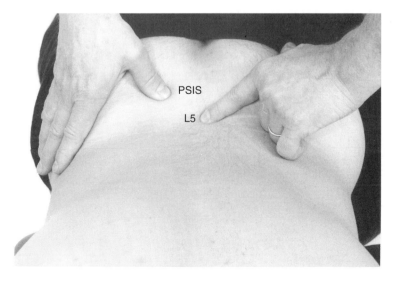

Fig. 3.15

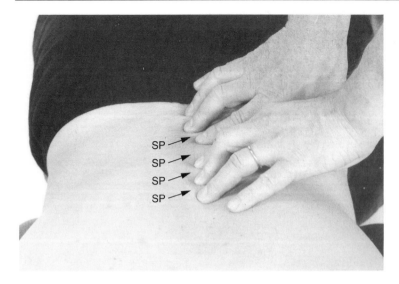

Fig. 3.16

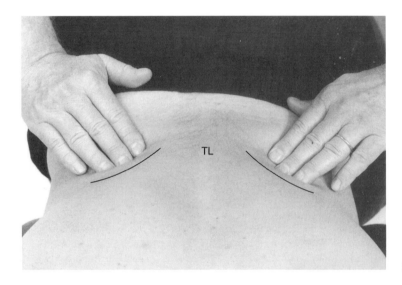

Fig. 3.17

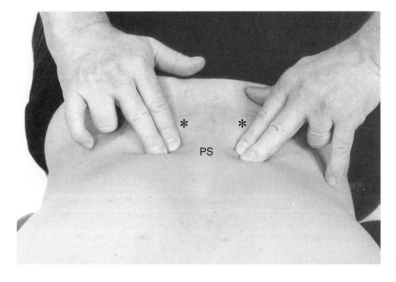

Fig. 3.18

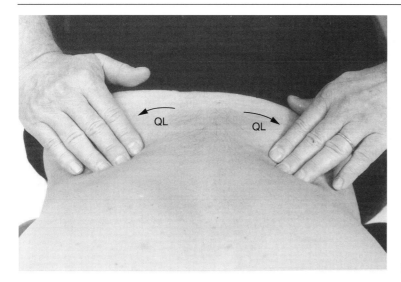

Fig. 3.19a

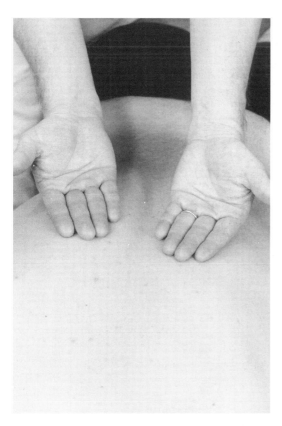

Fig. 3.19b

Palpation should be symmetrical with equal pressure bilaterally. Start superficially and then proceed to palpate deeper into the para-spinal musculature (PS). The aim is to detect symmetry or any specific palpable differences between the two sides. The objective is to determine the overall texture and tissue consistency. Palpation should be systematic in order to cover all regions. Maintain good posture throughout.

ii) Next reproduce Figure 3.18 by palpating more laterally in the region of the quadratus lumborum (QL) /external oblique muscles bilaterally, appreciating the bilateral consistency and texture of the soft tissues first superficially and then deeper into the tissue (Figure 3.19a). Take care to palpate equally maintaining posture and relaxed hands and arms. Try to visualize the structures immediately under the palpating fingers. Note any specific differences between the two sides. In this position also assess the bilateral temperature of the superficial skin and overlying soft tissues using the posterior or dorsum of the hands. Move the hands over a wide range bilaterally from the pelvic region and throughout the thoracolumbar region to the cervicothoracic junction (Figure 3.19b).

iii) Continue to palpate cephalad both superficially and deeper to include the lumbosacral soft tissue region bilaterally (Figure 3.20). Palpation should also include the region just medial to the PSIS and the sacroiliac joints (SI) bilaterally. Note the soft tissue consistency over this bony region (*).

iv) Continue to palpate along the pelvic crests bilaterally and in a lateral direction to determine the consistency of the soft tissues and drop down over the iliac crests bilaterally and appreciate both the superficial and deep texture of the gluteal muscle groups (GM) (Figure 3.21). This should include the gluteus medius and the gluteus maximus. Note the consistency of the soft tissue both superficially

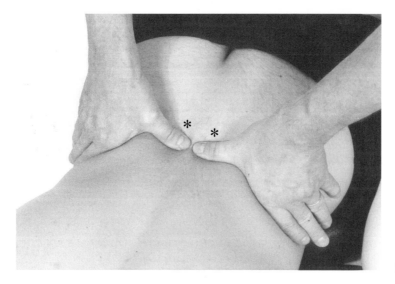

Fig. 3.20

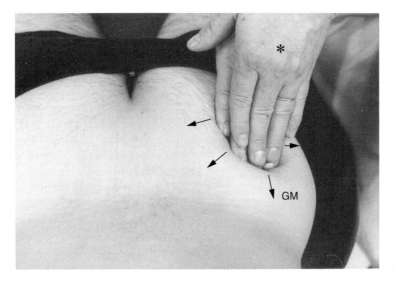

Fig. 3.21

and then deeper and always compare bilaterally. Note the posture of the palpating hands in a reinforced posture (*).

STATIC JOINT PLAY ANALYSIS

Assessing the presence or absence of inherent joint function such as joint play or spring of the lumbosacral and sacroiliac joints is an important aspect of the clinical assessment of patients with non-specific mechanical back pain. This procedure is performed with the patient in the prone posture with both the pelvis and lumbar spines supported and slightly flexed in order to expose the spinous process as palpable landmarks. This should be performed systematically beginning at the SI region and proceeding

cephalad to include the thoracolumbar spines. All skills should be practised and developed on both sides of the body in order to develop clinical flexibility. These skills will be introduced and transferred to other regions of the spine and the extremity joints in subsequent chapters.

Sacroiliac joints — posterior-anterior (P-A)

PSIS contact

i) Standing in a 45 degree fencer stance (from either side of the table), place both hands bilaterally over each PSIS with the calcaneal (heel) aspect of each hand (fleshy hypothenar eminence). The hands are slightly arched to accommodate the contour of the pelvic structures (Figure 3.22). Both arms should be straight and firm but not locked in extension. The sternal notch should be placed over the centre of the hands in the region of the sacral tubercles (*). This ensures equal distribution of weight prior to joint play procedures.

ii) Plantar flex the rear foot and bring the body weight over the midline. Apply a light but firm P-A force through the shoulder/arm along the line of the SI joint, first on the left and then the right (Figure 3.23). The application of joint play force should be oscillatory in nature in order to assess the natural joint compliance. The applied force should be equal on both sides and should be tolerated by the patient. Joint play direction should be along the joint line in a lateral and anterior direction towards the table (*). Ensure that assessment is performed on both sides to ensure some degree of consistency.

Sacral contact

i) Standing in the fencer stance position, as in Figure 3.23, place the thenar aspect of each hand over the sacral alar region bilaterally (just medial to the PSIS and slightly superior to S2 tubercle). Apply a firm oscillatory P-A joint spring challenge along the line of the SI joint in an anterior and lateral direction (Figure 3.24). Notice the heel of the hands are fairly close together for this exercise and depending on the size of the palpator's hands will determine whether both hands are initially contacting the sacral region. Note that the arms are firmly locked at the elbow and stabilized by the shoulder musculature (*).

LUMBAR SPINE – POSTERIOR-ANTERIOR JOINT PLAY ANALYSIS

i) Standing in a fencer stance on the left side of the patient locate the L4 spinous process (SP) as previously described above in Figure 3.12. Place the distal finger pads of the 1st, 2nd and 3rd fingers of the caudad (right) hand directly over the L4 and L5 SPs. The fingers should be pointing 45 degrees to the spine. The wrist should *not be* fully extended, but the hand should be flat against the soft tissue of the

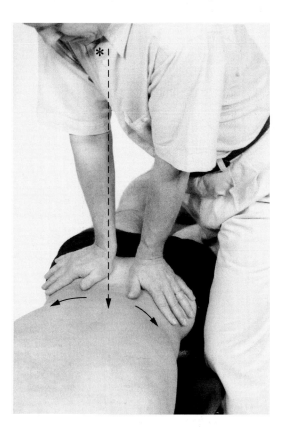

Fig. 3.22

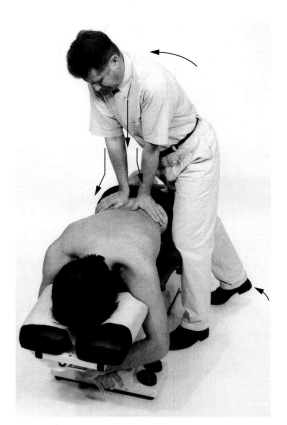

Fig. 3.23

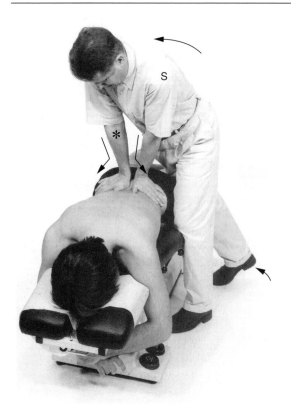

Fig. 3.24

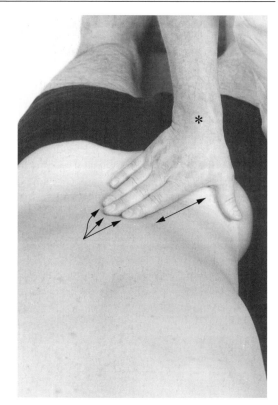

Fig. 3.25

paraspinal region (Figure 3.25) (*). (Note: the hands are interchangeable no matter what side of the body the practitioner is standing on.)

ii) Place the fingers of the cephalad hand (left) over the dorsum of the caudad hand (right) at a right angle in order that the 1st, 2nd and 3rd distal finger pads are contacting over the fingers of the right hand (Figure 3.26). Note the wrists are not fully extended to minimize the mechanical stress (*).

iii) Apply a firm P-A pressure through the L4/5 motion segment making sure the arms are straight and the force is generated through the shoulders and lower back, *not the hand contact* which is firmly placed over the spinal contact. Ensure that the sternal notch is directly over the contact hands (Figure 3.27). The normal springy compliance should be detected. The resistance should be elastic in nature keeping in mind the general orientation of the lumbar facet joints. Joint play force should be assisted by a simultaneous and coordinated movement of the lower limbs and pelvis by allowing the body weight to assist the joint play of the spinal structures (*). *The practitioner must be in a fencer stance position to be able to perform this skill.*

iv) Continue to assess the remaining lumbar motion segments and/or individual segments using the same procedure up to and including the thoracolumbar spinal region (Figure 3.28). Move cephalad in a systematic segment by segment fashion maintaining the fencer stance. *This P-A joint play analysis pattern can be extended to include all thoracic spine motion segments up to and including the cervicothoracic junction.*

v) An alternative hand contact using the hypothenar eminence with a reinforced hand, as above, may also be used and learned. The fleshy aspect of the left hypothenar eminence is placed over the spinous process of the mid-lumbar spine and reinforced with the other hand to support the contact (Figure 3.29). The support hand is slightly arched (*). This contact provides more give and force than the finger pad contact to be transmitted through to the spine. Assess for natural compliance during this assessment. The joint play assessment procedure should be repetitive and oscillatory in nature. Keep note of the sternal notch and fencer stance to maintain correct posture. Control the body drop through the front weight-bearing support leg to assist force production through the arms and hands into the spine.

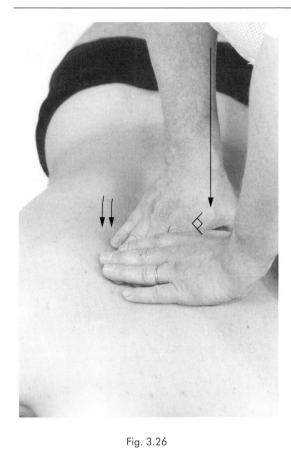

Fig. 3.26

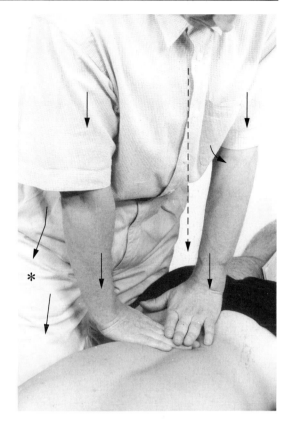

Fig. 3.27

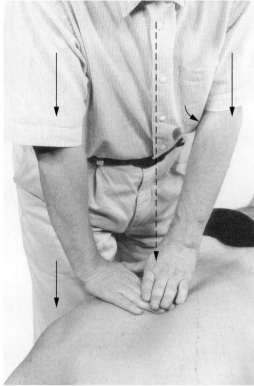

Fig. 3.28

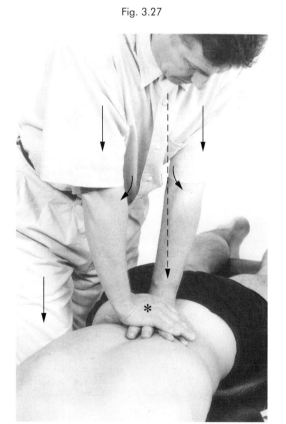

Fig. 3.29

vi) This alternate hand contact can also be used to assess P-A joint play into the thoracolumbar and thoracic spinal motion segments (Figure 3.30). The fencer stance must be maintained as the practitioner moves cephalad. Joint play force should be generated through the shoulders and pelvis with controlled body drop and transmitted into the hands to overcome the resistance at the spinal segment level.

LUMBAR SPINE – LATERAL TO MEDIAL JOINT PLAY ANALYSIS

i) Standing in a fencer or ski stance on the right side of the patient place the thumb pad of either hand on the lateral aspect of the spinous lamina junction of the L4 motion segment. Place the thumb pad of the other hand behind the contact thumb to reinforce the spinal position. Both hands should be in an arched posture to free the thumbs and accommodate the paraspinal soft tissue contour (Figure 3.31). In this case the thumb pad of the right hand is in contact with the spine. The thumb pad in contact with the spine should cover both spinous

processes and the interspinous space. The hands are completely in contact with the paraspinal region but the wrists are not hyperextended (*).

ii) Ensure that the thumbs are in direct contact with the skin overlying the spinous lamina junction and wrists are relaxed and slightly ulnar deviated which is a natural posture of the hand/wrist complex (Figure 3.32) (*).

iii) Apply a firm lateral to medial (towards the spinal midline) joint play force through the reinforced thumb contacts using the arms/shoulders and ulnar deviation of the wrists to generate enough force to challenge the lumbar facets and overcome the tissue resistance (Figure 3.33). A normal elastic compliance should be appreciated. The joint play should be performed in an oscillatory fashion to appreciate the natural joint and tissue give.

iv) Continue to utilize this joint play analysis throughout the lumbar and thoracic spinal motion segments and learn to perform the skills on both sides of the patient (Figure 3.34). Maintain either a ski or fencer stance at all times, lean against the table to support body weight and be reminded to generate

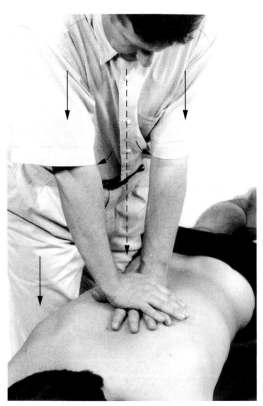

Fig. 3.30

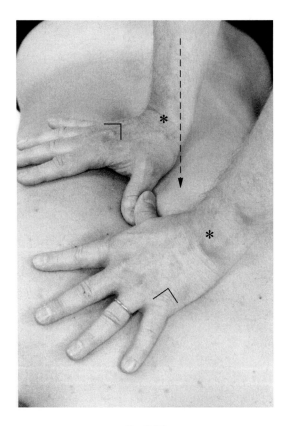

Fig. 3.31

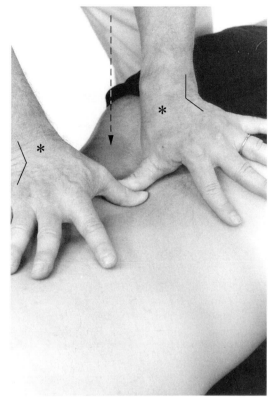

Fig. 3.32

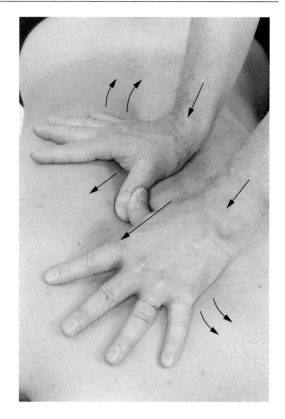

Fig. 3.33

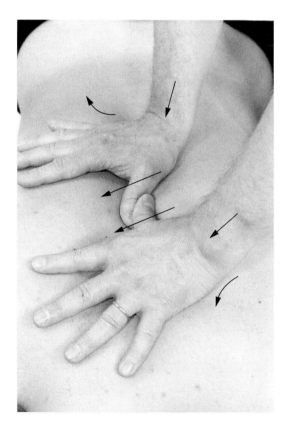

Fig. 3.34

necessary force through the shoulders and upper chest wall and not just the thumb contacts. Keep the sternal notch over the thumb contact to maintain correct body weight posture.

LUMBAR SPINE – COUNTER-ROTATION SPECIFIC JOINT PLAY ANALYSIS

i) Assume a fencer stance posture and place the thumb pad of the right hand at the spinous lamina junction of L3 and the thumb pad of the left hand at the spinous lamina junction of L4 (Figure 3.35). The thumbs are not in contact with the tip of the spinous process but more on the lateral edge. Both hands should adopt a firm but light chiropractic arch posture in order to accommodate the paraspinal soft tissue contour (*). Apply a firm lateral to medial joint play force simultaneously with both contact points using movement generated by the upper arm and chest wall. *Appreciate the joint give or compliance of a specific lumbar motion segment. The joint play is oscillatory in nature and repeated several times at each segment to appreciate the tissue resistance.*

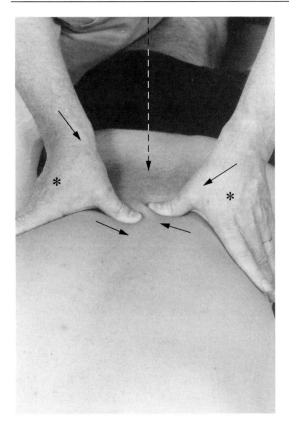

Fig. 3.35

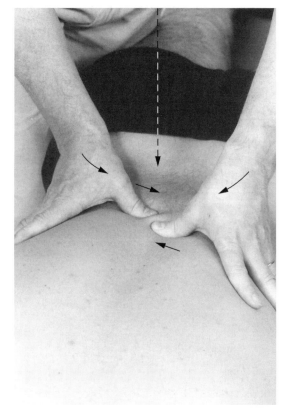

Fig. 3.36

ii) Switch the thumb contacts and repeat the lateral to medial joint play analysis in the opposite direction of a specific L3/L4 lumbar motion segment (Figure 3.36).

iii) The same skills may be used to assess one segment at a time by stabilizing one side and assessing joint play challenge with the other contact. The segment is stabilized by the thumb contact of the left hand (*) and the right thumb contact assesses joint play from lateral to medial against a fixed point (Figure 3.37). The joint play is oscillatory in nature and repeated several times at each segment.

iv) This specific analysis should be employed at all levels of the lumbar and lower thoracic spines in a comprehensive fashion. Ensure that all skills are learned from both sides of the table (Figure 3.38).

General rib spring – prone

i) Adopt a fencer stance posture with the patient in the prone position. Place the thenar and hypothenar eminences of each hand over the angle of the ribs with the fingers pointing lat-

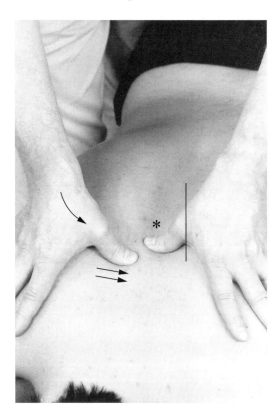

Fig. 3.37

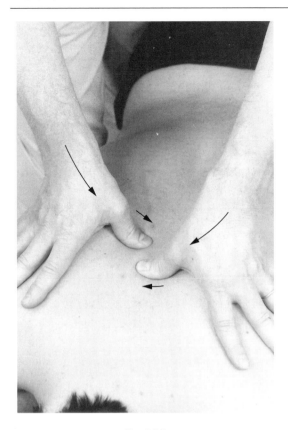

Fig. 3.38

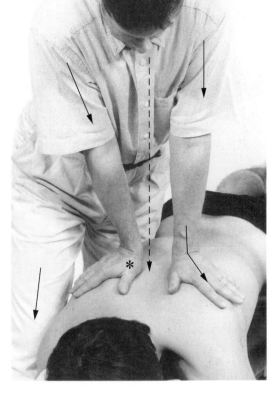

Fig. 3.39

erally and the hands arched over the rib contour (Figure 3.39). Ensure that the sternal notch falls between both hand contacts. Stabilize one side (*) and then apply a P-A and lateral joint play force through the ribs. Test one side and then stabilize appropriately and joint play the other side. Maintain firm extended elbows and generate the force through the shoulders and by controlling body drop by way of the front leg of the fencer stance. Apply as much force as the tissue resistance dictates. Keep in mind the ribs are very flexible and caution is extended when learning to palpate their compliance. Remember it is the joint play of the costotransverse articulation that is clinically relevant.

DYNAMIC END PLAY ANALYSIS – PELVIS AND SPINAL SEGMENTS

Pelvic complex and sacroiliac joint – standing movement analysis

Movement palpation of the sacroiliac joints is a common procedure to assess mechanical dysfunction and guide manipulative intervention. Like most motion palpation procedures the sacroiliac joint suffers from the same lack of inter-practitioner consistency which sheds doubt upon its clinical utility. Nonetheless, sacroiliac joint motion analysis has developed a standardized method that supports further consideration. This is of importance as part of an overall multidimensional assessment format. The following skills are to be introduced and learned within the context of a comprehensive examination of the musculoskeletal system. These skills should be learned with the context of known sacroiliac joint mechanics and other supportive palpation methods, particularly those employed in a non-weight-bearing posture.

Lateral bending

i) Kneeling behind the patient, locate and place the thumb pads under the inferior aspect of the PSIS landmark bilaterally. The fingers of the hand should stabilize the hands in order to maintain an accurate contact by contacting the gluteal region just inferior to the pelvic crests (Figure 3.40).

ii) Ask the patient to bend sideways and move the hand down the lateral aspect of the thigh as far as possible. Maintain contact at all times and

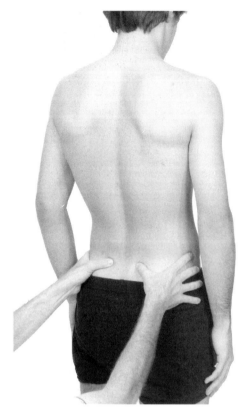

Fig. 3.40

assist the sideways movement of the pelvis. There is considerable sideways movement of the pelvis. In a normal situation both the PSISs and the pelvis generally should remain relatively level during full lateral bending indicating normal mechanical balance and the pelvis should sway and move in the opposite direction of lateral bending to balance the centre of gravity (Figure 3.41a). When the fingers do not remain level during lateral flexion possible clinical dysfunction may be present but needs to be confirmed by other clinical testing procedures (Figure 3.41b).

Reciprocal innominate movement

i) With reinforced thumb pads contacting the PSISs bilaterally, request a supported patient to flex one hip to 90 degrees. Under normal conditions, as the right hip is flexed the PSIS should drop posterior and inferior on the side of hip flexion and a reciprocal relative extension should take place on the stance side in order to balance the centre of gravity and overall pelvic mechanics (Figure 3.42).

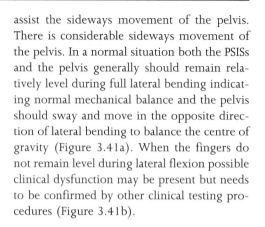

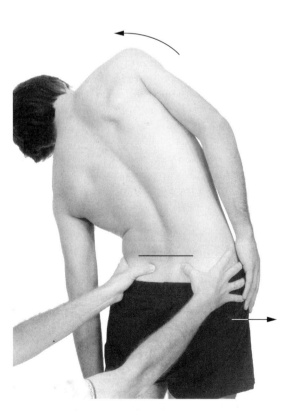

Fig. 3.41a

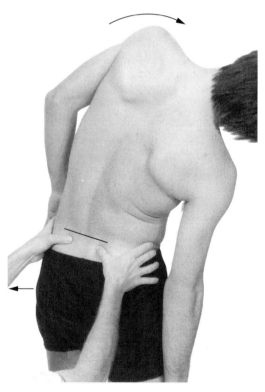

Fig. 3.41b

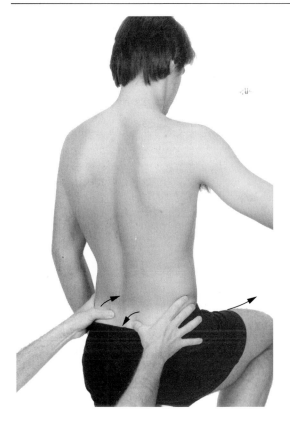

Fig. 3.42

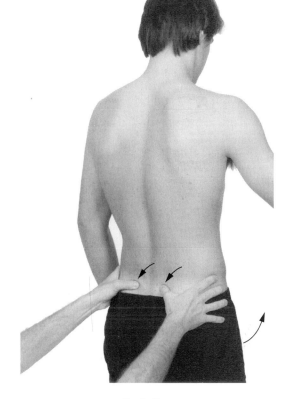

Fig. 3.43

ii) In a potential dysfunctional state both thumbs will move posterior and inferior with flexion of the right hip to 90 degrees indicating possible pelvic imbalance which requires further clinical investigation (Figure 3.43).

Specific sacroiliac joint movement palpation (nutation/counternutation – sacral base)

i) Contact one thumb under the inferior aspect of the PSIS and the other thumb is placed over the sacral ala which is located just superior and lateral to the 2nd sacral tubercle in the region of the 1st sacral segment (superior and medial to the PSIS) (*). Ensure that both palpation contacts are supported and firm (Figure 3.44).

ii) Ask the patient to flex the hip to 90 degrees. Observe a normal reciprocal movement of thumbs as the innominate flexes (PSIS posterior and inferior) and the sacral base moves anterior and inferior (nutation) (Figure 3.45). The movement is very subtle and very small in magnitude. The relative movement is

reflected through the soft tissue as the sacroiliac joint is deeply seated in the pelvic ring.

iii) If dysfunction is suspected the thumbs will move together (Figure 3.46). It must be kept in mind that these palpation procedures are only one aspect of any clinical assessment and must be placed in perspective with respect to their potential pathomechanical state. A number of other clinical tests combined with case history information assists in the clinical outcome and therapeutic intervention.

Specific sacroiliac joint movement palpation (innominate (ischial) flare)

i) With one thumb placed over the soft tissue covering the ischial tuberosity or just proximal to this point towards the sacral apex, place the left hand thumb midline on the sacral apex (Figure 3.47). Stabilize both palpating hands over the greater trochanter and pelvic brim. The right thumb is generally located equidistant between the greater trochanter and the sacral apex. This is the region of the ischial

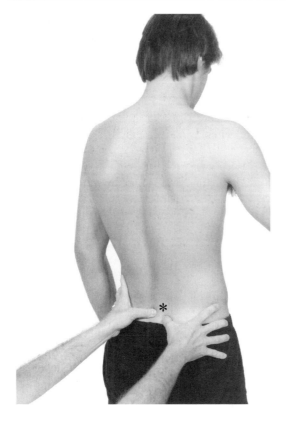

Fig. 3.44

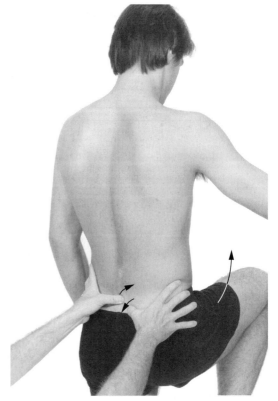

Fig. 3.45

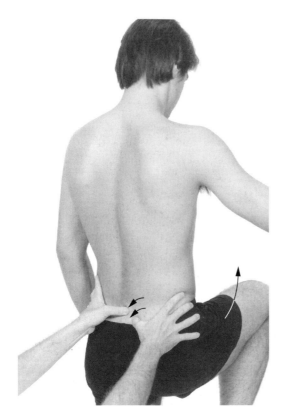

Fig. 3.46

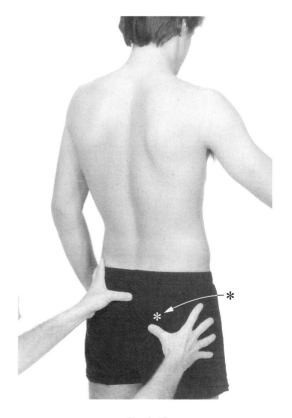

Fig. 3.47

tuberosity which is positioned very deep in the soft tissues of the gluteal region. The thumb contact should be light and superficial over the ischial tuberosity (*).

ii) Ask the supported patient to flex the hip and knee to 90 degrees. The ischial contact should move in a lateral and anterior direction following the line and natural contour of the sacroiliac joint. This is referred to as a 'J' motion of the innominate and is created by the anatomical angle of the sacroiliac joint (Figure 3.48). Care should be taken to ensure a firm but light contact over the tissue in order to follow the innominate movement.

iii) Dysfunction may be suspected when this motion is not accomplished and the movement is not symmetrical or full with no lateral anterior movement or 'J' motion noted (Figure 3.49). *Further clinical investigations would need to be performed to determine the nature and possible cause of this aberrant motion.*

Dynamic end play analysis of the thoracolumbar spine

Motion palpation of the lumbar spine has been shown to lack acceptable inter-rater consistency in a number of previously published studies (Hass and Panzer, 1995). Besides methodological flaws and inappropriate statistical analysis, palpation procedures were investigated in isolation which disregards typical clinical assessment protocols (Hass and Panzer, 1995). It may well be that the reliability of motion palpation is actually enhanced when combined with other typical clinical procedures such as palpation for bony and soft tissue tenderness (Keating et al., 1990). It has also been stated that the objectivity of motion palpation is improved when the procedures are standardized and based upon a consistent model and rationale (Byfield, 1997). With this in mind, it is the author's opinion that learning proficient motion palpation skills based upon a sound biomechanical model and joint kinematics is an important aspect of undergraduate skill learning. Therefore, the following section will focus on presenting motion palpation of the thoracolumbar spinal joints employing end play or end feel concepts as described by Peterson and Bergmann (1993). These palpation skills are designed to assess integrity of the elastic barrier or elastic zone of the joint.

Standardization should also include adhering to kinematic characteristics with respect to the area of

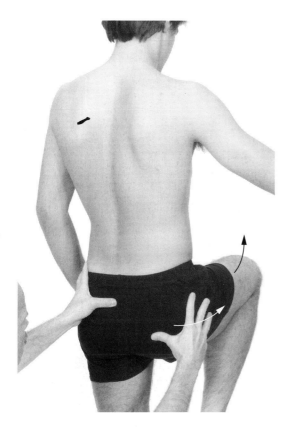

Fig. 3.48

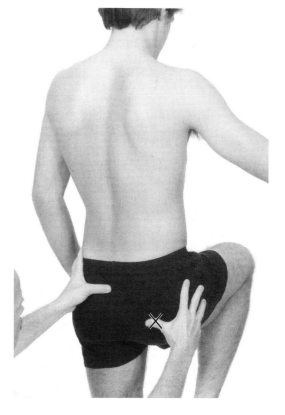

Fig. 3.49

the spine being assessed. This naturally requires that the palpator needs to become familiar with the functional anatomy and the known movement representative of the joints being examined. This should enhance specific psychomotor skills acquisition. It should also eliminate extraneous palpation procedures that are not required in a particular region of the spine that does not demonstrate all planes and axes of motion. Therefore, end play skills for the lumbar spine will focus on those axes of motion that are typical for that region of the spine. This is mainly for practical purposes to eliminate excessive movements that may not give additional information and aggravate the patient's presenting symptoms. In the lumbar spine it is recommended that rotation, lateral bending and combined rotation, lateral bending and extension movements be assessed. Flexion has been eliminated even though it is a primary motion in the lumbar spine as it is difficult to control patient's trunk weight while sitting and tension in the posterior ligament system during flexion may confound palpation procedures.

End play is defined as the assessment of the elastic barrier of a spinal joint at the end of the passive range of motion prior to paraphysiological space (Peterson and Bergmann, 1993). This particular aspect of joint function is clinically important to assess the functional integrity of the holding elements of the joint. Loss of end play, pain and local tenderness are considered important clinical findings related to a manipulable lesion (Peterson and Bergmann, 1993). Identifying the level and understanding the local and regional kinematics assist in deciding the type of manipulative intervention.

End play is a qualitative term to describe the natural compliance of spinal joints and related holding elements. The palpator needs to develop kinaesthetic skills as well as a strong biofunctional model to underpin clinical rationale (Peterson and Bergmann, 1993).

These concepts are transferable to all regions of the spine, as the joints are similar in nature. Therefore the clinical concepts of end play are similar in all regions.

Recommended sitting spinal palpation position

i) The standard palpation posture is performed with both practitioner and patient in the seated posture preferably using a specifically designed palpation stool. The practitioner sits off centre and close behind the patient with the left arm draped around the patient's shoulder (Figure 3.50). It is recommended that the

practitioner employ an adjusting table if a specific palpation stool is not available.

ii) The stabilizing arm (left) grips the bulk of the trapezius (*) with one hand and the other side of the shoulder with the flexor portion of the forearm (**) (Figure 3.51). This positioning permits easy access to the spinous processes on the ipsilateral side when palpating and provides a degree of control for the practitioner. Note that the practitioner sits close to the patient in order to control patient movement and keep the palpating levers to a minimum.

iii) Movement and control of the patient is then accomplished pulling and pushing the shoulder in order to introduce movement in the thoracolumbar spines with ease and efficiency (Figure 3.52). Note the proximity of the practitioner to the patient for ease of palpation (*) and the palpating arm/hand is tucked in close to the practitioner's body to assist end play and reduce leverage (**).

Lateral bending end play – lumbar spine

i) Sitting on the left side of the patient with the left arm stabilizing trunk movement, place

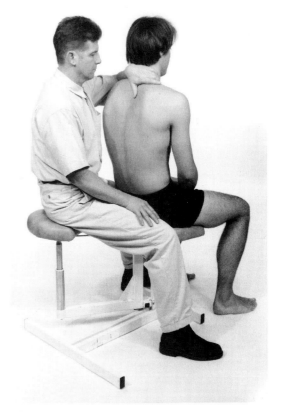

Fig. 3.50

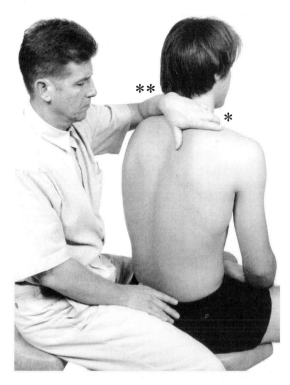

Fig. 3.51

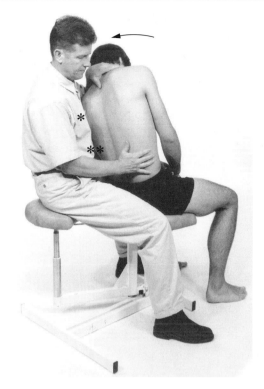

Fig. 3.52

the thumb pad of the right hand on the ipsilateral aspect of the spinous lamina junction of L4 (Figure 3.53). Ensure that the palpating hand is placed in a chiropractic arch posture in order to accommodate the lumbar paraspinal musculature (*). Make sure that the contact is an individual spinous process and not on the tip of the spinous process, but more on the lateral aspect in order to generate appropriate leverage.

ii) Pull the patient toward the practitioner laterally bending the lumbar spine fully and maintain firm contact on the spinous lamina junction of L4. When the spine is fully laterally flexed apply an end play counter movement in the opposite direction in order to assess the elastic components of the L4/L5 motion segment in lateral bending (Figure 3.54). The end play force should be generated from the shoulder of the practitioner in an oscillatory motion at the end of the range of motion (*) and not just by way of the thumb contact. The normal end play compliance should be pain free and elastic in nature. Continue to assess the remaining lumbar segmental levels employing the same end play palpation skills up to and including the thoracolumbar spinal

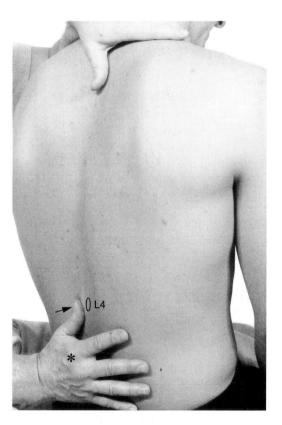

Fig. 3.53

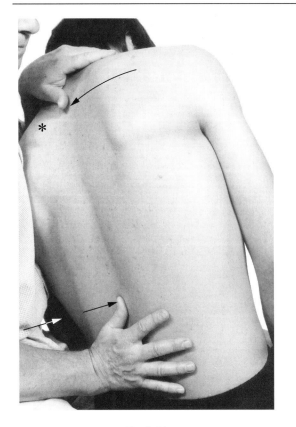

Fig. 3.54

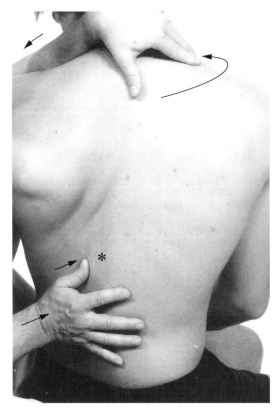

Fig. 3.55

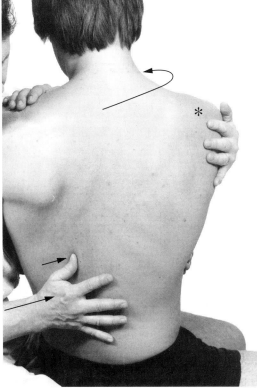

Fig. 3.56

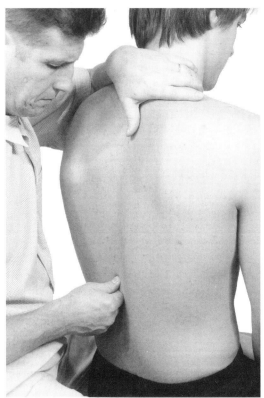

Fig. 3.57

motion segments up to and including the cervicothoracic segmental junction. Ensure that palpation is uniform and inclusive.

Rotation end play – lumbar spine

i) Begin with the patient seated and stabilized as in Figure 3.51. Contact the ipsilateral spinous lamina junction of L4 using the thumb pad of the right hand. Ensure that the contact hand is arched and fully contacts the skin and paraspinal musculature. Rotate the patient fully towards the practitioner in order to engage the elastic barrier or end play of the lumbar motion segment (Figure 3.55). Apply end play pressure at the full rotation or at patient's tolerance (*). Use an oscillatory end play technique.

ii) Continue to employ this rotational end play skill at all lumbar levels comparing each level and ensure that palpation is accomplished on both sides of the spine. An alternative support contact can be employed depending on the patient. Instead of contacting over the shoulder region the practitioner reaches around and grasps the patient's opposite arm in the triceps region to stabilize the trunk (Figure 3.56) (*). End play palpation is employed at the end of left posterior rotation to assess the elastic barrier of the spinal segment. These techniques can be used throughout all thoracolumbar spinal segments.

Extension end play – lumbar spine

i) Secure the patient in standard palpation posture as depicted in Figure 3.51, except in this instance sit more directly behind the patient. Place the thumb pad of the palpating hand directly over the spinous process of the thoracolumbar spine. Support the thumb with the index finger and wrap the other fingers into the hand (Figure 3.57).

ii) Gently pull the patient into extension and simultaneously apply forward movement of the palpation hand at end range. At this point assess end play compliance with a series of oscillatory movements in a posterior to anterior direction (Figure 3.58). Maintain the palpation arm close to the body and apply the end play pressure through the entire upper limb in order to generate sufficient forces (*). Continue to apply extension end play throughout the entire lumbar and thoracic spines.

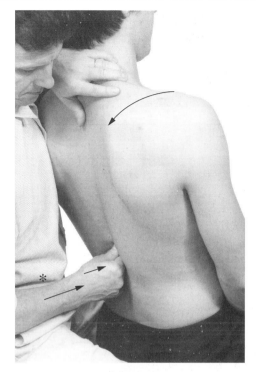

Fig. 3.58

Combined movement end play – lumbar spine

The lumbar spine has specific kinematic characteristics that should dictate examination procedures. With this in mind it would be clinically appropriate to combine various ranges of motion. This would economize time and simulate natural movements. It is the author's opinion that additional information is not necessarily gained by palpating in all planes and axes of motion.

i) Sit behind the patient and adopt the standard palpation posture securing the patient with the left arm around the patient's shoulder. Sit to one side in order to control the patient's body weight and movement. The palpation stool helps to maintain correct posture plus patient comfort and control. Place the thumb of the palpating hand on the ipsilateral side of the spinous lamina of L4 with the hand skilfully forming an arch configuration. Draw the patient towards the palpator at a 45 degree angle to introduce *rotation, extension and lateral bending* in one simultaneous movement (Figure 3.59). Apply an oscillatory end play pressure at the end of the patient's capable range of motion (*). Keep the palpating arm close to the body in order to restrain the levers to a minimum and reduce fatigue (**).

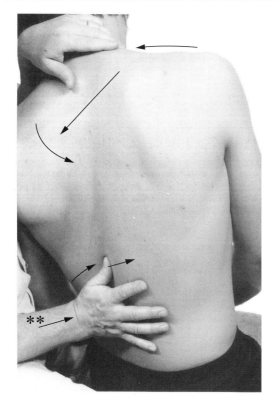

Fig. 3.59

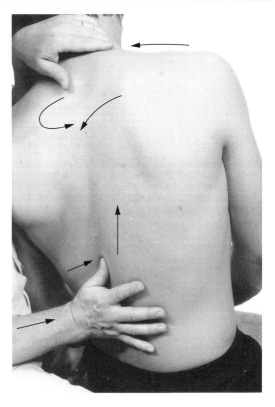

Fig. 3.60

ii) Continue to end play analyse the entire lumbar spine incorporating the thoracolumbar spinal region comparing each level and ensure that both left and right sides are palpated in exactly the same fashion (Figure 3.60).

SUMMARY

This chapter has presented a number of basic palpation skills required by the manual therapist in order to identify segmental dysfunction. The chapter focused on anatomical landmark location and fundamental motion palpation analysis skills commonly used by chiropractors. Though these particular skills are reported to demonstrate considerable variation within the various professions, the author has concentrated on isolating the basic psychomotor procedures. A sound biofunctional rationale has also underpinned these skills with respect to joint function and segmental imbalance.

Like all psychomotor skills these procedures need to be practised and developed over a significant period of time during both undergraduate and postgraduate professional growth.

REFERENCES

Byfield, D. (1996) *Chiropractic Manipulative Skills*. Butterworth-Heinemann, Oxford.

Byfield, D.C.M. (1997) Investigation of motion palpation of the spine using mechanical models. MPhil Thesis, University of Southampton.

Hass, M., Panzer, D.M. (1995) Palpatory diagnosis of subluxation. In: *Foundation of Chiropractic Subluxation* (Gatterman, M. ed.). pp. 56–67. Mosby, Toronto.

Hubka, M.J. (1994) Palpation for spinal tenderness: a reliable and accurate method for identifying the target of spinal manipulation. *Chiro Tech*. **6**, 5–8.

Keating, J.C., Bergmann, T.F., Jacobs, G.E., Finer, B.A., Larson, K. (1990) Interexaminer reliability of eight evaluative dimensions of lumbar segmental abnormality. *J Manipulative Physiol Ther*. **13**, 463–470.

Peterson, D.H., Bergmann, T.F. (1993) Joint assessment principles and procedures. In: *Chiropractic Technique* (Bergmann, T.F., Peterson, D.H., Lawrence, D.L., eds). pp. 51–122. Churchill Livingstone, London.

FURTHER READING

Bergmann, T., Peterson, D., Lawrence, D. (1993) *Chiropractic Technique*. Churchill Livingstone, London.

Magee, D. (1987) *Orthopaedic Physical Assessment*. W.B. Saunders Company, London.

4

Basic thoracic spine palpation and landmark identification skills

Stuart Kinsinger

Palpation of the thoracic spine with reference to specific anatomical landmarks and soft tissue configurations is a learned skill requiring many hours of practice and concentration. This is also a very important region from a clinical perspective. Therefore, a strong basic anatomical knowledge must be established prior to embarking upon learning these psychomotor skill sets with any degree of proficiency. It has also been reported that visual and mental imagery may enhance complex psychomotor skill learning. Following appreciation of various structural markers, the next step is to introduce standard palpation protocols to analyse the static and dynamic qualities of the spinal and pelvic articulations. Lack of articular movement has been identified as a principal chiropractic tenet and a fundamental requirement prior to spinal manipulative intervention. This analysis is underpinned by a descriptive theory outlining the active and passive range of motion of diarthroidial joints. It also classifies which particular holding elements (capsular and ligamentous) are challenged during each specific palpation procedure, permitting the clinician to establish a reasonably accurate segmental diagnosis. The procedure should identify which aspect of the joint range of motion is impaired (active, passive, joint play, end play), the intersegmental level and potential pain generators.

This chapter will focus on landmark identification and two types of joint assessment: joint play and end feel (play). These are rudimentary joint analysis techniques and play an important role in establishing a clinical diagnosis in chiropractic practice. Joint play is described as the natural compliance of a joint in its neutral position. End feel (play) is the assessment of the quality of the elastic barrier of the joint at the extent of the passive range prior to the paraphysiological space. Joint play is performed in the neutral static posture while end play is performed at the end of the normal range of motion of a joint challenging the important support structures. This chapter will also focus on appropriate postural skills for the practitioner when learning and performing these basic palpatory skills for the thoracic spine region. This chapter will also present a variety of soft tissue palpation techniques plus identification of a number of important anatomical landmarks in the thoracic region. Learning an efficient posture during this initializing period will provide the framework for more complex psychomotor skills implemented later during undergraduate education.

The chapter will cover a number of areas including:

- Soft tissue palpation and identification skills
- Anatomical landmark palpation and identification skills
- Joint play analysis skills

Note: At all times students must practice their postural skills while working at their palpation skills. These were introduced during the lumbar spine and sacroiliac joint regions and should be reinforced during all palpation procedures.

ANTERIOR CHEST WALL PALPATION

i) With your partner lying comfortably supine, use one or two fingers to palpate the episternal notch of the manubrium (the upper border of the sternum(*)) located in between the origin of each sternocleidomastoid (SCM) muscle (Figure 4.1). Also feel slightly laterally to each side for the sternoclavicular joint space and then back to the episternal notch.

ii) Using both hands move inferiorly to palpate the transverse ridge of the manubriosternal junction which is located at the level of the 2nd rib anteriorly (*) (Figure 4.2).

iii) Move the inferior hand down to the lower border of the sternum palpating the overall structure and the individual costosternal joints located at the lateral edge of the sternum (*). Continue to palpate inferiorly to the xiphoid (Figure 4.3). Gently move superiorly from the lower end to palpate the xipho-sternal ridge, which may be difficult to appreciate.

iv) From the lower end of the sternum move out laterally and inferiorly down to feel the costochondral cartilages which coalesce to join the sternum. You should be able to differentiate the cartilaginous and osseous structures including the distal ends of the ribs as they angle down to the costochondral region (Figure 4.4). With your partner's consent, use one or both hands to palpate those ribs that articulate directly with the sternum, ribs 1 to 6. This requires careful palpation considering the palpation zone.

v) From the medial aspect at the sternocostal joints trace laterally with your fingertips along the shaft of each rib as the rib bends posteriorly around the thorax (Figure 4.5). The first rib disappears under the clavicle and is not usually palpable. Also be sure to feel the soft intercostal muscles between the ribs.

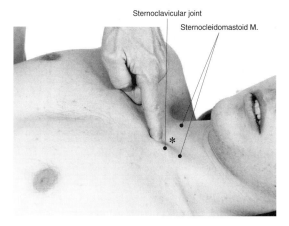

Fig. 4.1

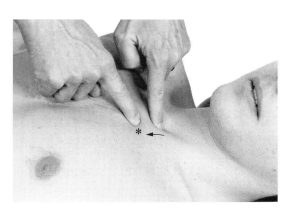

Fig. 4.2

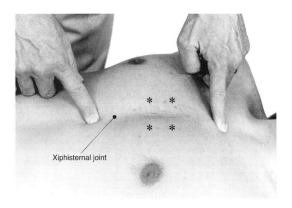

Fig. 4.3

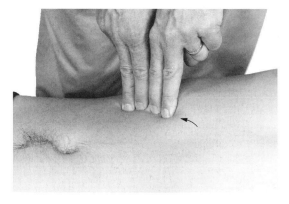

Fig. 4.4

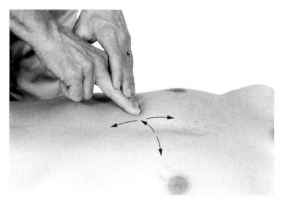

Fig. 4.5

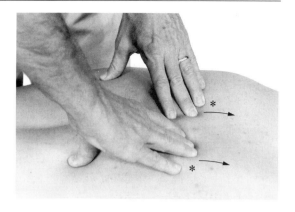

Fig. 4.8

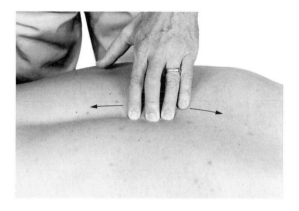

Fig. 4.6

POSTERIOR SPINAL PALPATION

i) With your partner lying face down, start by using the finger pads from one hand to identify, count and palpate the individual vertebral spinous processes (Figure 4.6). This should be all the way from the lower neck at the cervicothoracic junction down to the sacral tubercles. Ensure that you identify the individual levels using the spine of the scapula, the inferior pole of the scapula and the angle of the ribs to assist spinal level location.

ii) Use two or more finger pads and other palpating combinations, continue to feel the spinous processes (Figure 4.7) with the interspinous spaces, above and below. Press gently in the interspace feeling the elastic give of the interspinous ligament.

iii) Now using the fingertips of both hands palpate the adjacent paraspinal muscles bilaterally (Figure 4.8). Attempt to assess general muscle bulk, tone and texture from the upper thoracic to the sacroiliac region. Assess the quality of the paraspinal muscle groups in the different regions of the spine. Move laterally out over the angle of the rib to include the entire paraspinal region (*).

iv) Palpate the paraspinal muscles that run from just above the gluteal area to the thoracolumbar junction spine (Figure 4.9). These are clinically important structures and should be included in all examination procedures.

v) By moving the finger pads or thumb pads 1–2 cm out from the midline (1.0–1.5 finger breadth) feel for the transverse processes (TVP) by pressing firmer and deeper into the tissue (Figure 4.10a). The TVPs are very difficult structures to palpate and appreciate. They

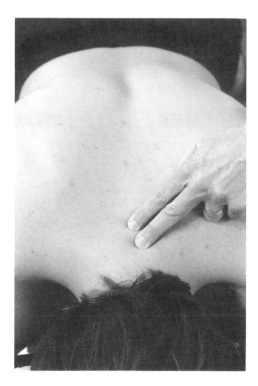

Fig. 4.7

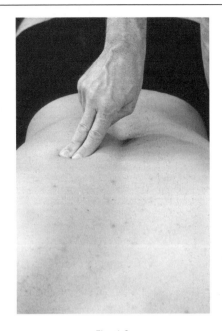

Fig. 4.9

are located deep under the paraspinal tissue and constitute a very important manipulative lever. Try to visualize the structures while you are palpating, but try not to second guess yourself. The palpator may use either the thumbs or the *index/middle fingers* to palpate these structures.

- For the upper thoracic spine (T1–T4) the TVP is located *one interspinous space* above the target spinous process (Figure 4.10b).
- For the midthoracic spine (T5–T9) the TVPs are located *two interspinous spaces* above the target spinous process (Figure 4.10c).
- For the lower thoracic spine (T10–T12) the TVPs are located *one interspinous space* above the target spinous process (Figure 4.10d).

vi) Move both hands down and place the side of each hand and the index finger along the lowest ribs (*) reaching up to place the thumbs on

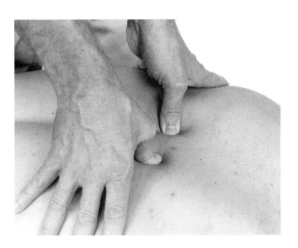

Fig. 4.10a

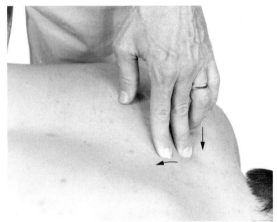

Fig. 4.10b

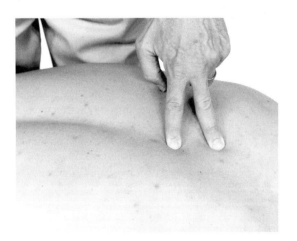

Fig. 4.10c

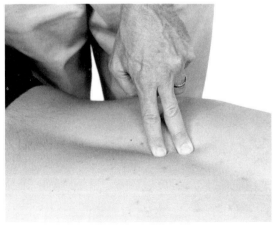

Fig. 4.10d

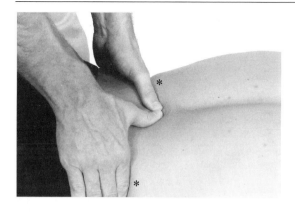

Fig. 4.11

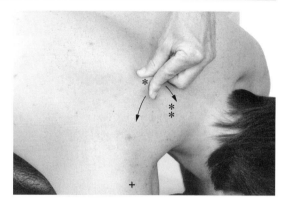

Fig. 4.12a

the spinous process of the thoracolumbar junction (T12–L1) (Figure 4.11). Bring the thumbs together to locate this region of the spine. This region of the spine is also a very important region clinically from a mechanical pain perspective.

LANDMARK PALPATION OF THE SCAPULAR REGION

Spine of the scapula

With your partner face down, locate the 3rd thoracic spinous process and palpate laterally to find the medial border of the scapula, at which point you should be able to find the spine of the scapula (*) (Figure 4.12a). This demarcates the supraspinous fossa from the infraspinous fossa. Continue to palpate laterally along the spine of the scapula to the acromion at the AC joint (+). If you palpate superiorly from the spine of the scapula along the medial border of the scapula you should be able to define the superior border of the scapula (**).

The spine of the scapula may also be palpated using three fingers to appreciate the osseous structures including the acromion (Figure 4.12b).

Inferior pole of the scapula

i)   Palpate inferiorly along the medial border of the scapula appreciating the contour and shape until the inferior pole is reached where both the medial and lateral borders meet (Figure 4.13). This should be at the level of the spinous process of T7 or T8 (*).

ii) Now palpate both superior (*) and inferior angles (**) simultaneously to appreciate the size of the scapula (Figure 4.14a). Continue to palpate the structures surrounding the sca-

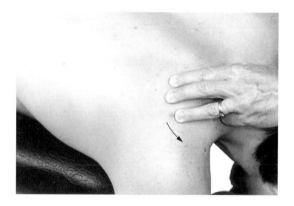

Fig. 4.12b

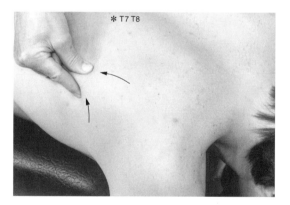

Fig. 4.13

pula at this point, particularly the soft tissues, primarily the supraspinatous (*), infraspinatous (**), teres major (+) and teres minor (Figure 4.14b).

iii) Extend your partner's arm back to lie along the table or place the dorsum of the hand in the lower back region and observe the scapula retract from the thorax making all these landmarks more prominent for your palpation (Figure 4.15).

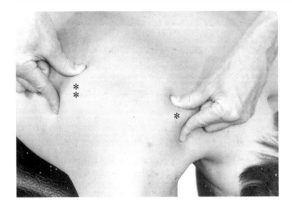

Fig. 4.14a

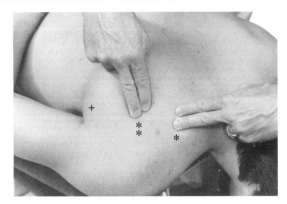

Fig. 4.14b

SUMMARY

This chapter has presented an overview of the palpation methods required to locate major anatomical landmarks of the thoracic spine. A basic introduction to a variety of fundamental joint play procedures and joint assessment skills has also been presented. It is up to the student to pursue acquiring and developing these skills as a prerequisite to advancing their training to include various manipulative psychomotor skills that are introduced later in the educational curriculum.

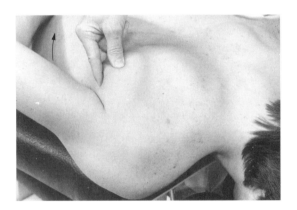

Fig. 4.15

FURTHER READING

Bergmann, T., Peterson, D., Lawrence, D. (1993) *Chiropractic Technique.* Churchill Livingstone, London.

Byfield, D. (1996) *Chiropractic Manipulative Skills.* Butterworth-Heinemann, Oxford.

Magee, D. (1987) *Orthopaedic Physical Assessment.* W.B. Saunders Company, London.

5

Basic cervicothoracic and occiput palpation and landmark identification skills

Stuart Kinsinger

Palpation of the cervicothoracic spine with reference to specific anatomical landmarks and soft tissue configurations is a learned skill requiring many hours of practice and concentration. This is also a very important region from a clinical perspective. Therefore, a strong basic anatomical knowledge must be established prior to embarking upon learning these psychomotor skill sets with any degree of proficiency. It has also been reported that visual and mental imagery may enhance complex psychomotor skill learning. Following appreciation of various structural markers, the next step is to introduce standard palpation protocols to analyse the static and dynamic qualities of the spinal and pelvic articulations. Lack of articular movement has been identified as a principal chiropractic tenet and a fundamental requirement prior to spinal manipulative intervention. This analysis is underpinned by a descriptive theory outlining the active and passive range of motion of diarthroidial joints. It also classifies which particular holding elements (capsular and ligamentous) are challenged during each specific palpation procedure, permitting the clinician to establish a reasonably accurate segmental diagnosis. The procedure should identify which aspect of the joint range of motion is impaired (active, passive, joint play, end play), the intersegmental level and potential pain generators.

This chapter will focus on landmark identification and two types of joint assessment: joint play and end feel (play). These are rudimentary joint analysis techniques and play an important role in establishing a clinical diagnosis in chiropractic practice. Joint play is described as the natural compliance of a joint in its neutral position. End feel (play) is the assessment of the quality of the elastic barrier of the joint at the extent of the passive range prior to the paraphysiological space. Joint play is performed in the neutral static posture, while end play is performed at the end of the normal range of motion of a joint challenging the important support structures. This chapter will also focus on appropriate postural skills for the practitioner when learning and performing these basic palpatory skills for the cervicothoracic spine region. This chapter will also present a variety of soft tissue palpation techniques plus identification of a number of important anatomical landmarks in the cervicothoracic region. Learning an efficient posture during this initializing period will provide the framework for more complex psychomotor skills implemented later during undergraduate education.

The chapter will cover a number of areas including:

- Soft tissue palpation and identification skills
- Anatomical landmark palpation and identification skills
- Joint play analysis skills.

SITTING PALPATION

i)   A number of structures are both visible and palpable on the anterior aspect of the neck including the anterior scalenes and the sterno-cleidomastoid (SCM) (Figure 5.1). Also note the attachment of these myofascial structures onto the clavicle and first rib (*). These structures should be palpated bilaterally (**) and also note the angle of the jaw as a reference point.

ii) Standing behind the patient palpate the anterior neck musculature with a very light touch from your fingertips. Slight resistance to neck rotation with the right hand while palpating with the left hand makes these muscle fibres quite prominent (Figure 5.2). Trace the full length of the SCM from the mastoid to the sternoclavicular (*). Palpate bilaterally.

iii) Now move to the TMJ (temporomandibular joint), and use one finger to palpate the posterior condyle just in front of the tragus of the ear (Figure 5.3). You should be able to appreciate the posterior ridge of the condyle (*).

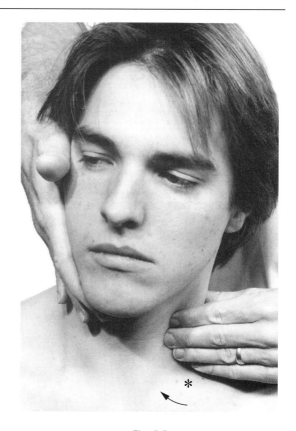

Fig. 5.2

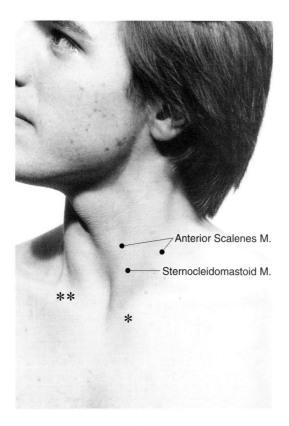

Anterior Scalenes M.

Sternocleidomastoid M.

**

*

Fig. 5.1

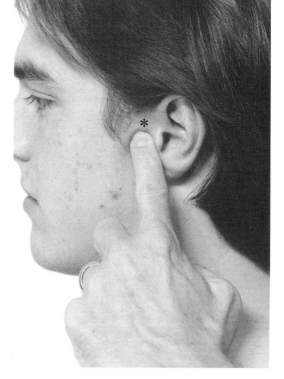

*

Fig. 5.3

iv) Use two fingers to feel the motion of the TMJ. Place the middle finger just anterior to the index finger over the anterior and posterior aspects of the condyle of the mandible (*). Ask your partner to open and close the mouth and appreciate the movement of the condyle as it moves back and forth within the mandibular fossa (Figure 5.4). This joint has important clinical significance for a number of common presentations.

v) Palpate the prominent mastoid process posterior to the pinna of the ear (Figure 5.5). This is the origin for the SCM. A number of structures can be accessed from this position including the lateral occipital rim which functions as an attachment point for the large posterior cervical postural musculature (*). Also note the prominence of the SCM (**) and the upper trapezius (***).

vi) Move posteriorly and medially to the midline of the cervical spine. Begin palpation at the suboccipital region in the midline and palpate down the central cervical spine to the first large prominent spinous process of C7 after C2 that is also known as the vertebral prominens. In order to ensure the level place the

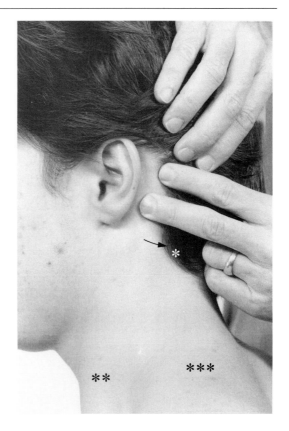

Fig. 5.5

index finger at C6–C7 interspinous space and flex the head and neck forward (Figure 5.6a). The space should increase. As you extend the patient's head and neck the space should decrease and the spinous process of C6 should slide forward (Figure 5.6b). This should be appreciated by the index finger (*). The C6 is the last movable segment due to the stabilizing influence of the attachment of the first rib at the C7 level and functions as an important clinical landmark for manipulative therapists.

LANDMARK PALPATION IN THE PRONE POSITION

i) Begin by locating the mastoid process landmark directly posterior to the earlobe (Figure 5.7). Just inferior and either anterior or posterior to the mastoid process is the TVP of atlas (C1) (*). This segment has some clinical significance as a number of mechanical syndromes are related to dysfunction of the occiput/atlas/axis segmental region. By palpating forward from the TVP of C1 the pal-

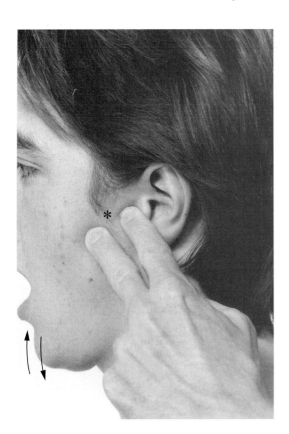

Fig. 5.4

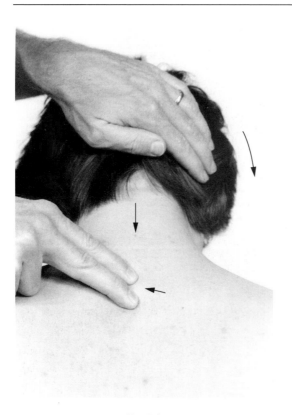

Fig. 5.6a

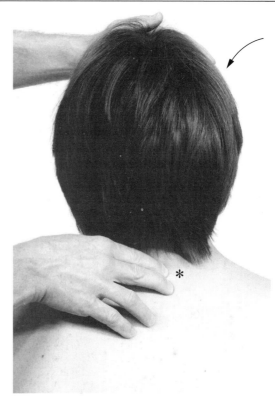

Fig. 5.6b

pator should locate the angle of the mandible (**).

ii) From this location move medially along the suboccipital ridge using the index and middle palpating fingers to the midline of the occipital rim (*) (Figure 5.8). The occipital rim is the attachment point for a number of important postural extensor muscles including the

splenius capitus, semispinalis capitus and the spinalis capitus. This region also plays an important clinical role in headache and other mechanical pain conditions.

iii) Once the palpator has reached the midline simply proceed in a cephalad direction and locate the external occipital protuberance (EOP) (*) (Figure 5.9).

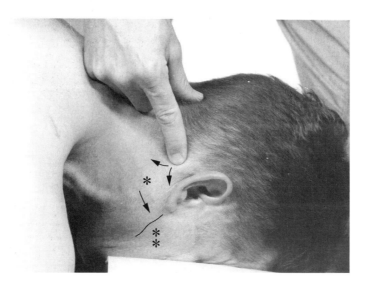

Fig. 5.7

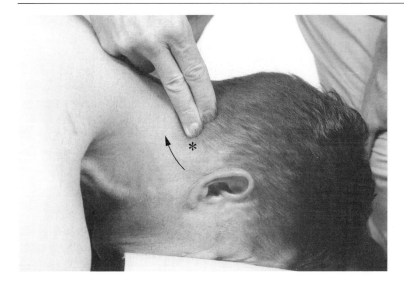

Fig. 5.8

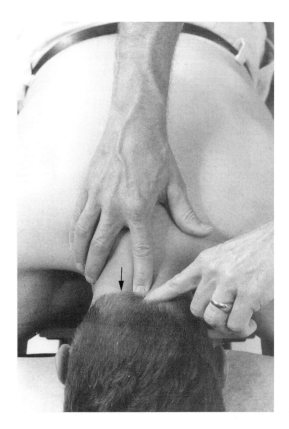

Fig. 5.9

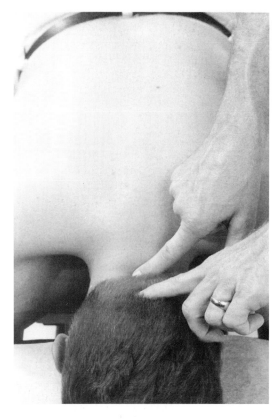

Fig. 5.10

iv) From the EOP, moving inferiorly, the next palpable midline structure is the large spinous process of C2 approximately 3 cm below the EOP (Figure 5.10). The posterior arch of atlas (C1) is located between these two structures and is usually difficult to feel by palpation.

v) Changing contacts, use both thumbs and trace the suboccipital ridge on each side from the mastoid to the EOP and back (Figure 5.11).

vi) Drop the headpiece forward slightly to flex the cervical spine. Now use thumb and finger pads of the first and middle fingers to locate and appreciate the posterior cervical spine, parti-

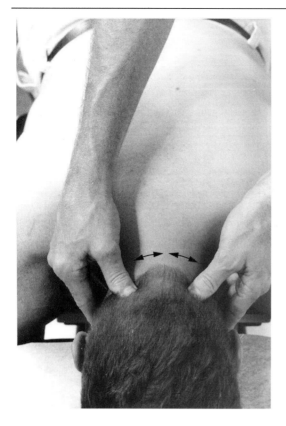

Fig. 5.11

cularly the cervical articular pillars bilaterally (Figure 5.12). Begin at the suboccipital region and work your way down to the CT junction. The pillars are tiny structures but important from a clinical perspective as they demarcate the posterior joints of the spine so often responsible for mechanical neck pain. Now add a very light posterior to anterior (P-A) push to the articular pillars to appreciate the joint play of the cervical joints. By moving your palpating fingers laterally about 2 finger breadths you will feel the TVPs (*). They are extremely small and tender and act as muscle attachment points on each side of the neck. You may have to push slightly more firmly to identify the articular ridge.

vii) Identify the midline landmarks at both ends of the cervical spine: the EOP and the C7 spinous process (Figure 5.13). Also observe the general contour of the neck and upper thoracic spine noting the shape, symmetry and contour of the overall muscle structures.

viii) At this point continue to palpate down the thoracic spine identifying various spinal levels and appreciating related soft tissues (Figure 5.14).

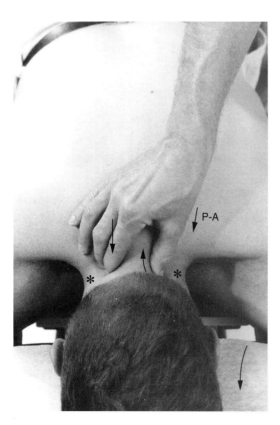

Fig. 5.12

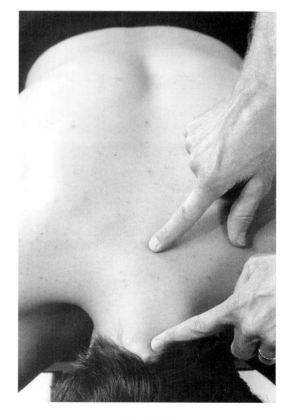

Fig. 5.13

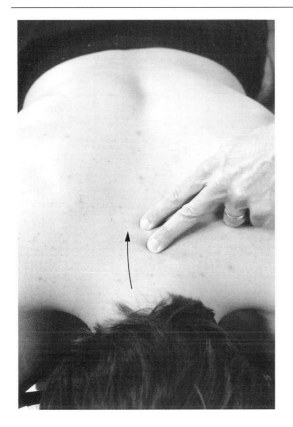

Fig. 5.14

SUMMARY

This section has presented an overview of the palpation methods required to locate major anatomical landmarks of the cervicothoracic spine and occiput. A basic introduction to a variety of fundamental joint play procedures and joint assessment skills has also been presented. It is up to the student to pursue acquiring and developing these skills as a prerequisite to advancing their training to include various manipulative psychomotor skills that are introduced later in the educational curriculum.

FURTHER READING

Bergmann, T., Peterson, D., Lawrence, D. (1993) *Chiropractic Technique*. Churchill Livingstone, London.

Byfield, D. (1996) *Chiropractic Manipulative Skills*. Butterworth-Heinemann, Oxford.

Magee, D. (1987) *Orthopaedic Physical Assessment*. W.B. Saunders Company, London.

6

Landmark location and palpation skills for the lower extremity

David Byfield

INTRODUCTION

Palpation of the lower extremity with reference to specific anatomical landmarks and soft tissue configurations is a learned skill requiring many hours of practice and concentration. This is also a very important region from a clinical perspective, particularly in many sports-related injuries. Therefore, a strong basic anatomical knowledge must be established prior to embarking upon learning these psychomotor skill sets with any degree of proficiency. It has also been reported that visual and mental imagery may enhance complex psychomotor skill learning. Following appreciation of various structural markers, the next step is to introduce standard palpation protocols to analyse the static and dynamic qualities of the articulations of the lower extremity. Lack of articular movement has been identified as a principal chiropractic tenet and a fundamental requirement prior to manipulative intervention. This analysis is underpinned by a descriptive theory outlining the active and passive range of motion of diarthroidial joints. It also classifies which particular holding elements (capsular and ligamentous) are challenged during each specific palpation procedure, permitting the clinician to establish a reasonably accurate diagnosis of dysfunction. The procedure should identify which aspect of the joint range of motion is impaired (active, passive, joint play).

This chapter will focus on landmark identification and passive joint play assessment. These are rudimentary joint analysis techniques and play an impor-

tant role in establishing a clinical diagnosis in chiropractic practice. Joint play is described as the natural compliance of a joint in its neutral or end range position.

This chapter will also focus on appropriate postural skills for the practitioner when learning and performing these basic palpatory skills for the lower extremity. This section will also present a variety of soft tissue palpation techniques plus identification of a number of important anatomical landmarks for the major articulations of the lower extremity. Learning an efficient posture during this initializing period will provide the framework for more complex psychomotor skills implemented later during undergraduate education.

Injuries to the articulations of the lower extremity are common. It is therefore important for the undergraduate to develop a working knowledge of the functional anatomy and joint mechanics of all major extremity articulations in order to provide management and care for these clinical conditions. Furthermore, the foot and knee are very complex multijoint structures that are subject to overuse and asymmetrical mechanical loading during the performance of a number of common activities. This places additional stress on the associated soft tissue and ligamentous holding elements contributing to various pain syndromes. Clinical management and subsequent rehabilitation are dependent upon accurate clinical assessment of the pain producing structures and a clinical impression to guide management.

The process begins early during undergraduate training that includes reasonably accurate anatomical landmark location of the extremity joints, related structures and associated soft tissues. It is also important to begin appreciating active and passive ranges of motion of extremity joints plus the differences related to the quality of their clinical significance.

This chapter will introduce hard and soft landmark location of the foot/ankle, knee and hip joints of the lower extremity. The chapter will also demonstrate a number of rudimentary passive joint play procedures for the major joints of the lower extremity. This will introduce the student to appreciate normal extremity joint play and begin to develop the skills of joint analysis. It is also advisable to learn to visualize the anatomical structures when palpating and locating various landmarks. It is reported to enhance the learning experience.

Section 1 The foot and ankle

Section 1 will cover the foot/ankle complex

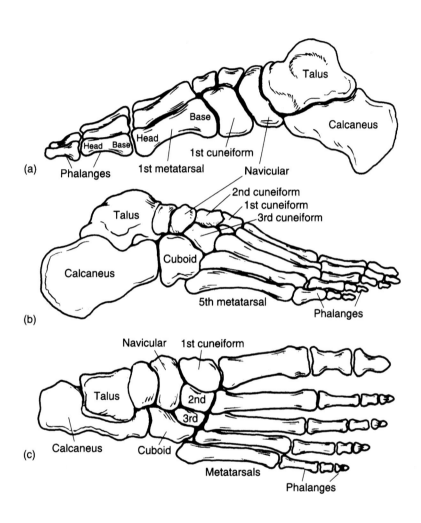

ACTIVE RANGE OF MOTION AND LANDMARK LOCATION

i) It is important to stabilize the ankle/foot complex during palpation assessment procedures. Sit at the end of the table and support the foot in the palm of the hand with the fingers wrapped around the calcaneus to control foot motion and posture (Figure 6.1). This frees the opposite hand to palpate the structures of the foot/ankle complex. The practitioner's support arm is resting on the left thigh adding more control.

ii) With the foot/ankle supported, a general assessment of the overall range of motion can be performed: dorsiflexion (DF) and eversion (E) (Figure 6.2a) and plantar flexion (PF) and supination (S) (Figure 6.2b). This accommodates more complex combined movements of the rear foot. These movements can be quickly assessed to appreciate the gross foot/ankle movement capabilities. Note the stabilizing hand and the ease of examination.

iii) Begin landmark palpation on the medial side of the foot. Stabilize the foot with the left hand and palpate with the right hand on the patient's right foot (Figure 6.3). Note the palpator's support arm is resting on the thigh to

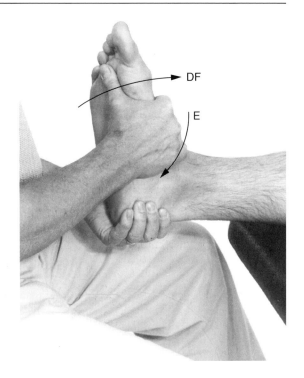

Fig. 6.2a

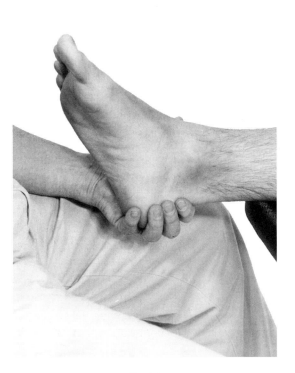

Fig. 6.1

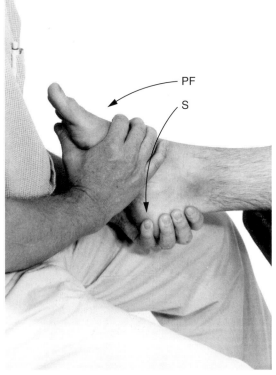

Fig. 6.2b

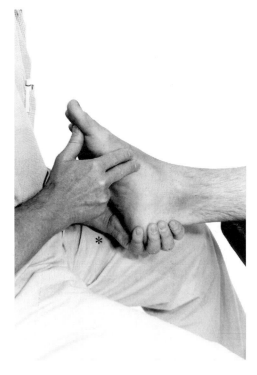

Fig. 6.3

reduce any strain during long examination procedures (*).

iv) Prior to palpating the foot it is recommended that a general visual observation of the foot/ankle be conducted to note any obvious abnormalities, always comparing left and right extremities (Figure 6.4). Take note of the non-weight-bearing medial, lateral and transverse longitudinal arches. Also observe for any swelling, discoloration or skin lesions.

MEDIAL ASPECT OF THE FOOT/ANKLE

Osseous landmarks

First metatarsophalangeal joint (MTP)

i) Position the foot as in Figure 6.3. Use the *right index and middle fingers or the thumb pad* to palpate the medial aspect of the first MTP joint beginning distally to proximal to locate the proximal end of the first phalanx as it articulates with the distal end of the first metatarsal (Figure 6.5). The joint space is very small and is distinguished by the broadening of the proximal and distal aspects of the first metatarsal and the proximal phalanx.

Metatarsals (MT)

i) Next probe along the shaft of the first metatarsal from the MTP joint using either the pal-

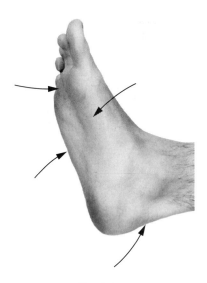

Fig. 6.4

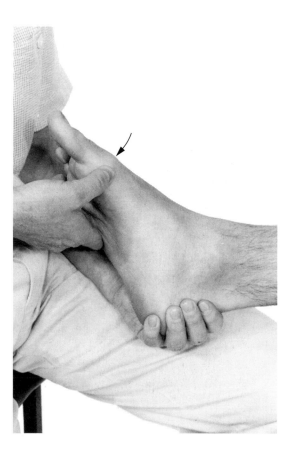

Fig. 6.5

pating fingers (Figure 6.6a) or the thumb pad to identify the structures (Figure 6.6b). This can extend into palpation of the other metatarsals going from medial to lateral across the dorsum of the foot.

First (medial) cuneiform

i) Continue to probe along the first MT using the finger pads and as it flares at the proximal end it articulates with the first cuneiform creating the first metatarsocuneiform joint (Figure 6.7a).

ii) Continue to interchange the finger pads with the palpating thumb to appreciate fully the structures and develop manual dexterity (Figure 6.7b). This is a flat joint and very small. Place the finger pads across the joint line and attempt to appreciate the joint space. Maintain stability of the foot during palpation to maximize findings. Also visualize the anatomical structures during palpation.

Navicular

i) Continue along the medial border of the foot and palpate the navicular tubercle that is described as a large bony prominence (Figure 6.8). The navicular is an important anatomical feature of the midfoot region as it articulates with several other structures including the cuneiforms distally(*) and the talus proximally (**).

Head of talus

i) The head of the talus is located directly proximal to the navicular and is optimally found with the foot in slight plantar flexion (Figure 6.9). The talus articulates primarily with the distal aspects of the tibia and fibula, navicular and the calcaneus. Eversion of the rear foot also assists location of the head of the talus. The talus is also found between the medial and lateral malleolli.

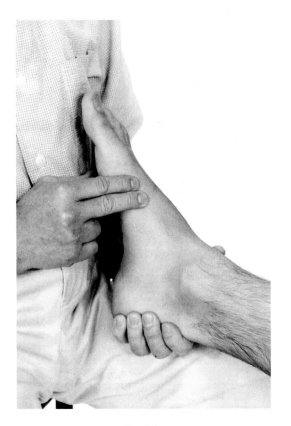

Fig. 6.6a

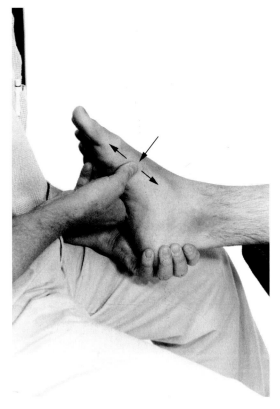

Fig. 6.6b

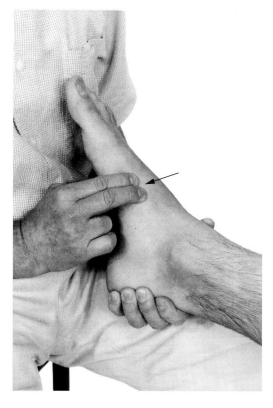

Fig. 6.7a

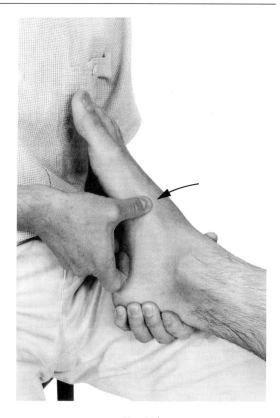

Fig. 6.7b

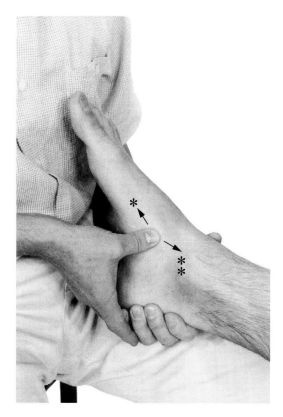

Fig. 6.8

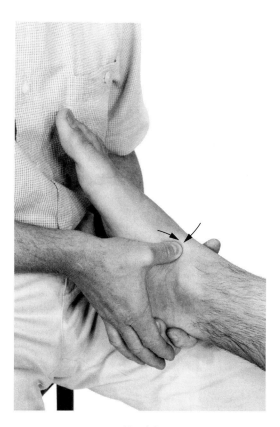
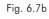

Fig. 6.9

Medial malleolus

i) Directly proximal to the head of the talus is the prominent medial malleolus which forms the most distal aspect of the tibia as it articulates with the talus (Figure 6.10a). Continue to visualize the structures during palpation and maintain stability of the foot with the opposite hand to ensure palpation accuracy. Palpate the inferior tip of the medial malleolus with the palpating thumb (Figure 6.10b).

Sustentaculum tali (ST)

i) Immediately below (plantarward) the medial malleolus (approximately one finger breadth) is the ST (Figure 6.11). The ST is a small outgrowth, which acts as an attachment point for the spring ligament which stabilizes the medial aspect of the ankle and has clinical importance.

Medial calcaneus

i) Directly posterior to the MM and the ST is the medial superior aspect of the calcaneus (Figure 6.12). The calcaneus is a large bone which makes up most of the heel structure of the rear foot and acts as an attachment for the Achilles tendon. There is a prominent fat pad on the underside of the heel to cushion weight bearing and the calcaneus tends to flare as you palpate posteriorly.

Achilles tendon insertion

i) Continue to palpate cephalad from the medial calcaneus and find the insertion of the Achilles tendon into the superior aspect of the calcaneus (Figure 6.13).

Achilles tendon

i) Continue to palpate cephalad and explore the entire Achilles tendon from the superior aspect of the calcaneus to the musculotendinous insertion at the gastrocnemius–soleus muscles. Dorsiflex the ankle to place the Achilles tendon under some stretch in order to identify and palpate with more accuracy (Figure 6.14). Use a pincher grip of the thumb and 1st digit to palpate the Achilles tendon.

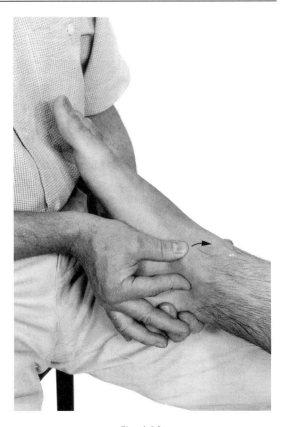

Fig. 6.10a

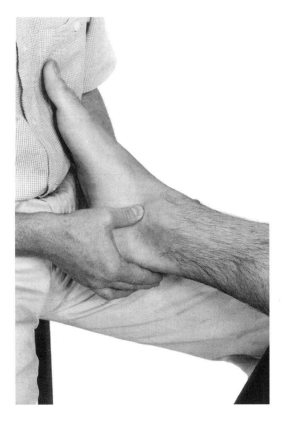

Fig. 6.10b

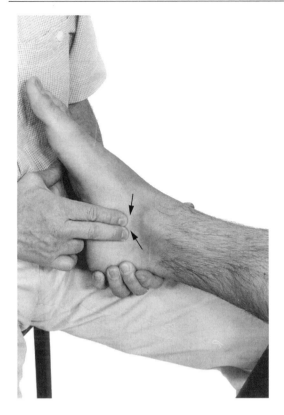

Fig. 6.11

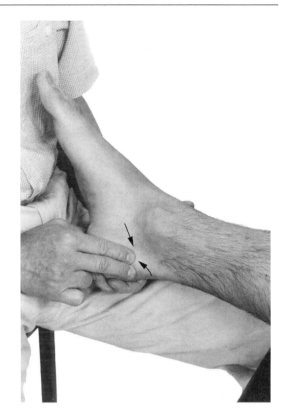

Fig. 6.12

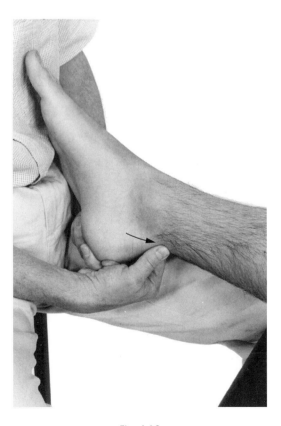

Fig. 6.13

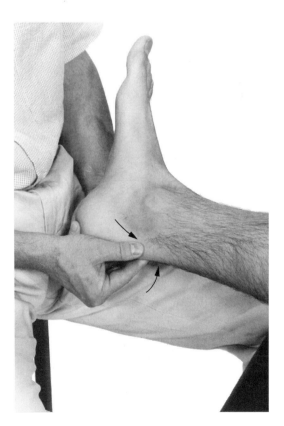

Fig. 6.14

LATERAL ASPECT OF THE FOOT

Superficial soft anatomical structures

i) Take note of some of the important superficial anatomical structures of interest on the dorsum and lateral aspect of the foot (Figure 6.15). Tibialis anterior (TA) tendon, extensor hallucis longus (EHL) tendon, extensor digitorum longus (EDL) tendons and extensor digitorum brevis (EDB) muscle belly.

ii) Note the osseous and soft tissue structures, particularly the peroneus longus (PL) and brevis (PB) tendons located inferior to the lateral malleolus (*) (Figure 6.16).

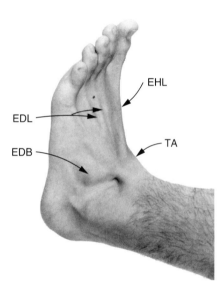

Fig. 6.15

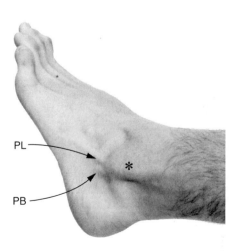

Fig. 6.16

Osseous landmarks

Fifth metatarsophalangeal joint (MTP)

i) In order to palpate the lateral aspect of the foot grasp the foot as in Figure 6.3 reversing the hands in order that the left hand is free to locate and palpate the various structures. The 5th MTP joint is found by palpating along the shaft of the phalanges until the base of the proximal phalanx flares (Figure 6.17).

Fifth metatarsal (MT) and styloid process (SP)

i) Continue to palpate laterally along from the 5th MTP joint, to include the 5th MT, to where it flares at the base to become the SP (Figure 6.18). Palpate into the depression on the proximal end of the styloid. The SP is a point of muscle attachment.

Cuboid

i) Directly proximal to and behind the SP lies the cuboid. It flares at the distal end near its articu-

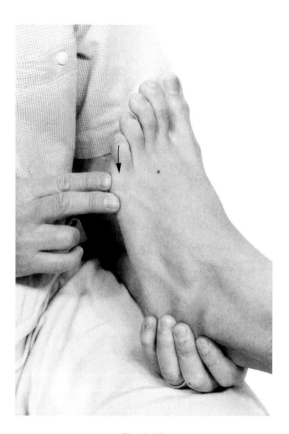

Fig. 6.17

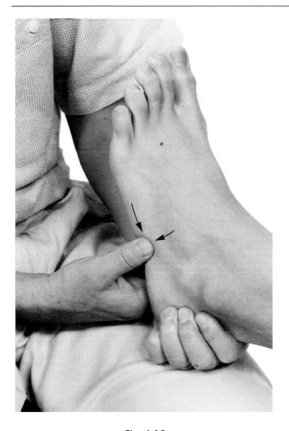

Fig. 6.18

lation with the SP and is characterized by a depression located in the middle of the structure (Figure 6.19). The tendon of the peroneus longus is situated here and has clinical significance.

Lateral aspect of calcaneus

i) Proximal to the cuboid is the lateral calcaneus which is characterized by the peroneal tubercle (Figure 6.20). Continue to palpate posteriorly as the calcaneus flares similar to the medial aspect.

ii) Grasp the posterior aspect of the calcaneus and palpate the region, assessing the insertion of the Achilles tendon (*) and the related soft tissue structures on the lateral aspect of the foot (Figure 6.21).

iii) Palpate more proximally to appreciate the large Achilles tendon structure with the foot plantar flexed in order to relax the tendinous fibres (Figure 6.22).

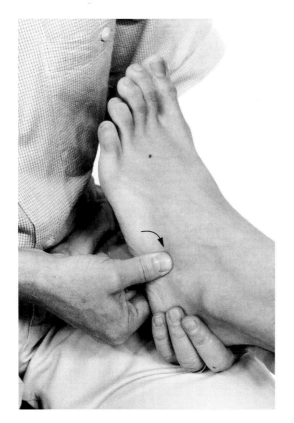

Fig. 6.19

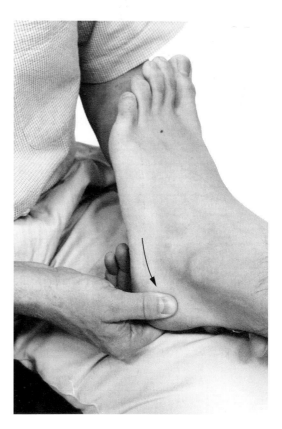

Fig. 6.20

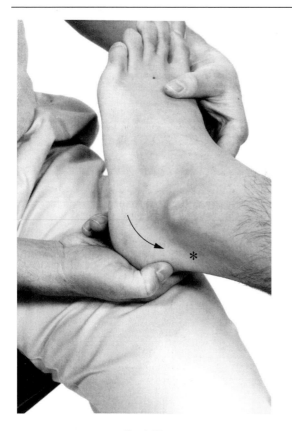

Fig. 6.21

Lateral malleolus

i) Directly above the calcaneus and distal to the Achilles insertion is the lateral malleolus which is the distal projection of the fibula (Figure 6.23). The lateral malleolus projects lower down than the medial malleolus. The inferior border of the lateral malleolus is the attachment point for a number of stabilizing ligaments which are implicated during inversion sprains. This region has a number of clinical implications.

ii) Locate the most anterior aspect of the lateral malleolus and plantar flex the foot. Just distal to this point in this position is the dome of the talus from the lateral side (Figure 6.24) (*).

iii) With the ankle joint in the neutral position palpate anterior to the lateral malleolus to locate the sinus tarsi region (Figure 6.25). This is a depression in the talus which houses the extensor digitorum brevis muscle.

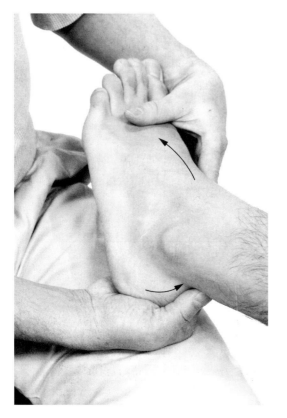

Fig. 6.22

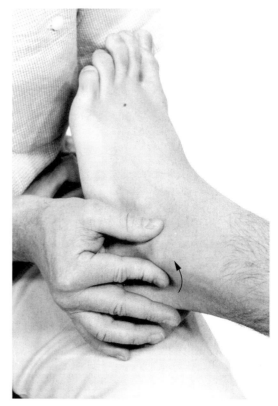

Fig. 6.23

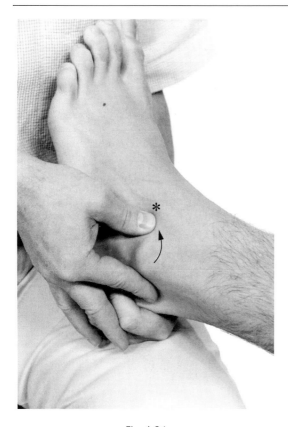

Fig. 6.24

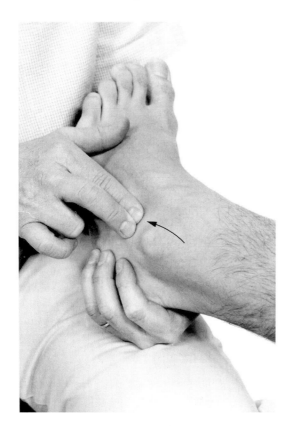

Fig. 6.25

PLANTAR ASPECT OF THE FOOT

i) Observe the plantar surface of the foot noting any callous formations, particularly along the metatarsal pads (*), which may indicate excessive wear and present some clinical significance and the heel/calcaneal region (**). Also observe the medial (M) and lateral (L) longitudinal arches for shape and contour (Figure 6.26).

ii) Support the dorsum of the foot with one hand and place the lower leg over the palpator's knee for added support. Dorsiflex the foot/ankle for ease of palpation and visual observation. Use the free hand to begin palpating the heel (*) and calcaneal region on the *medial aspect* of the plantar surface of the foot (Figure 6.27). This is the insertion of the broad plantar fascia which may have clinical significance.

iii) Palpate along the medial border (arch) palpating the inferior aspect of various structures already described from proximal to distal, including the navicular, cuneiforms and metatarsals up to and including the 1st MTP joint (Figure 6.28).

iv) Now begin to palpate from the medial plantar to lateral plantar aspect of the foot. Palpate the distal edge of the calcaneus as it broadens laterally (Figure 6.29). This is a common region for foot pain as a result of stress placed on the insertion of the plantar fascia (*).

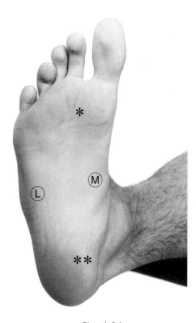

Fig. 6.26

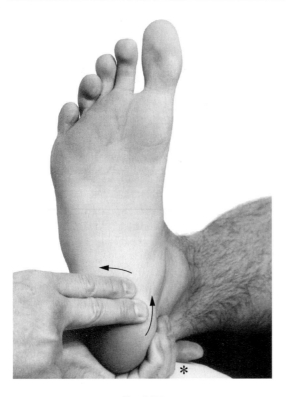

Fig. 6.27

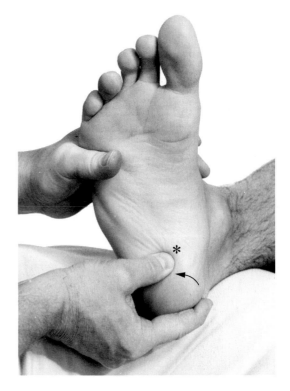

Fig. 6.29

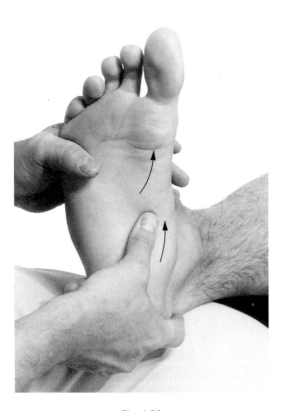

Fig. 6.28

v)   Palpate along the lateral border (arch) palpating the inferior aspect of various structures already described including the cuboid (Figure 6.30) (*).

vi) Next palpate laterally and continue distally to the styloid of the 5th metatarsal up to and including the 5th MTP joint from proximal to distal (Figure 6.31) (*). Keep the foot supported and dorsiflexed during the palpation exercise.

vii) Then continue to palpate distally along the metatarsal pads from lateral to medial to appreciate all the MTP articulations and associated soft tissues (Figure 6.32). Gently push the palpating thumb from inferior to superior to appreciate the flexibility and give offered by the MTP joints (*).

viii) Now dorsiflex the great toe and palpate for the two sesamoid bones located on the plantar surface of the 1st MTP joint (Figure 6.33) (*). These structures are buried in the fat pad of this region and provide extra leverage and tendon support during gait. This region has clinical significance in terms of foot pain and possible management strategies.

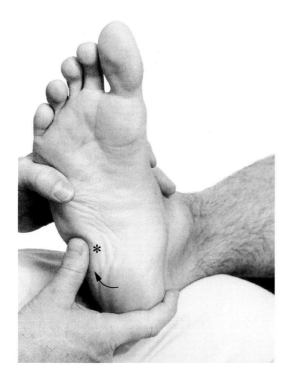

Fig. 6.30

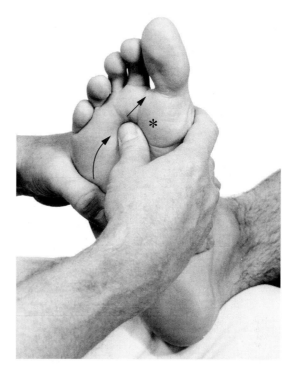

Fig. 6.32

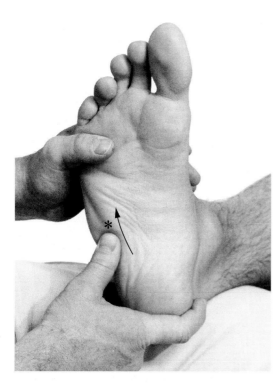

Fig. 6.31

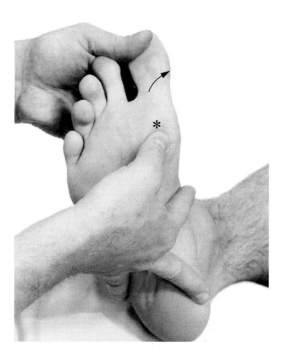

Fig. 6.33

Soft tissue landmarks

Extensor hallucis longus (EHL)(see Figures 6.15 and 6.16)

i) Support the foot as shown in Figure 6.3 and dorsiflex the great toe. Using the thumb pad of the opposite hand apply counterpressure over the dorsum aspect of the distal phalanx and note the large tendon sheath visible (Figure 6.34).

Extensor digitorum longus (EDL)

i) Support the foot as in Figure 6.3. Dorsiflex toes 2–5 and apply general counterpressure to the distal phalanges and note the tendon sheaths visible on the dorsum of the foot (Figure 6.35).

Peroneus longus (PL) and brevis (PB)

i) Evert the foot, stabilize the dorsum of the foot and apply counterpressure. Note the tendon sheaths around the inferior aspect of the lateral malleolus and wrapping over and under the midfoot region at the insertion points (Figure 6.36).

Tibialis anterior (TA)

i) Dorsiflex and invert the foot and apply counterpressure. Note the tendon sheath and the bulk of the muscle located in the anterior compartment of the lower leg (Figure 6.37).

Summary

i) Figure 6.38 demonstrates the important muscular structures related to the dorsum of the foot in a collective fashion.

Lateral collateral ligaments (LCL)

i) The important stabilizing ligaments on the lateral side of the ankle are located inferior, posterior and anterior to the lateral malleolus and can be generally palpated using both the thumb and 1st finger pad (Figure 6.39). Locating the ligaments is enhanced by invert-

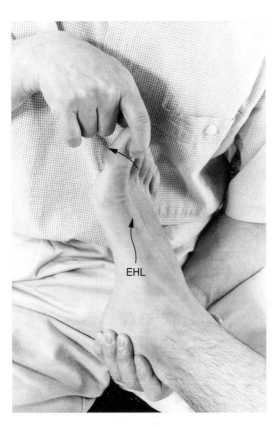

Fig. 6.34

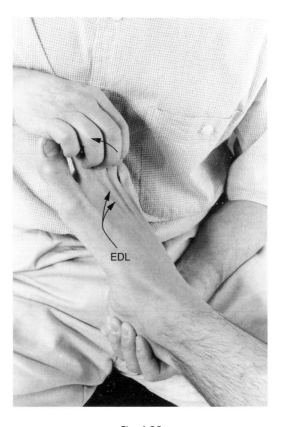

Fig. 6.35

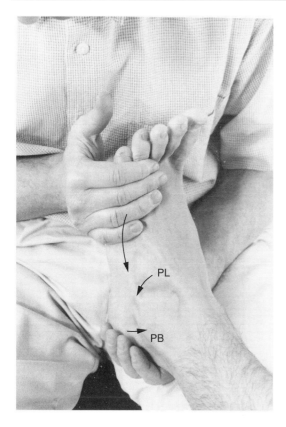

Fig. 6.36

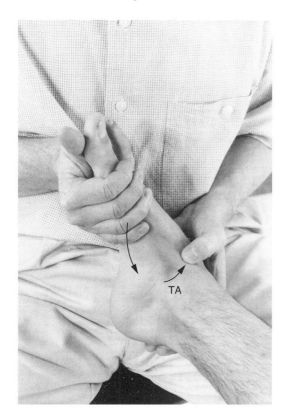

Fig. 6.37

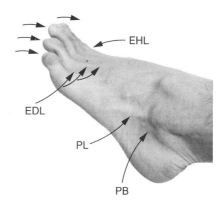

Fig. 6.38

ing and plantar flexing the foot. Two specific LCLs are shown below.

Anterior talofibular ligament (ATL)

i) Plantar flex and invert the foot. Palpate just distal to the anterior inferior aspect of the lateral malleolus towards the dome of the talus (Figure 6.40). This ligament structure has clinical significance with respect to commonly encountered inversion sprains.

Calcaneofibular ligament (CFL)

i) With the foot inverted and plantar flexed palpate just posterior to the inferior tip of the lateral malleolus for this ligament structure. As with the ATL, the CFL has important clinical significance regarding activity-related injuries to the ankle (Figure 6.41) (*).

Medial collateral ligament (MCL) (deltoid ligament)

i) This structure is palpable just inferior to the medial malleolus. The medial ligaments are thicker and stronger than the lateral and more difficult to locate. These ligaments may have clinical significance as a result of eversion sprains which are much less common than their inversion counterpart. Evert the foot/ankle when palpating this ligament (Figure 6.42).

Achilles tendon (AT)

i) Palpate the Achilles tendon with the 1st and 2nd digits, beginning at its insertion on the

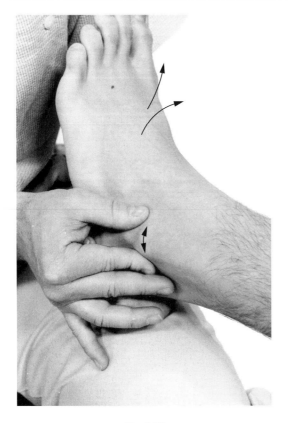

Fig. 6.39

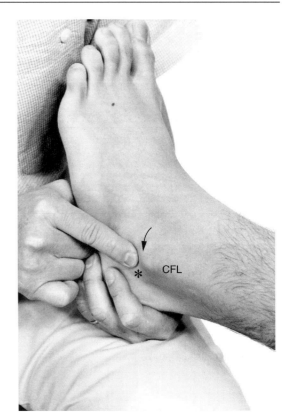

Fig. 6.41

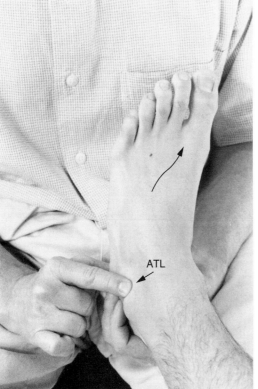

Fig. 6.40

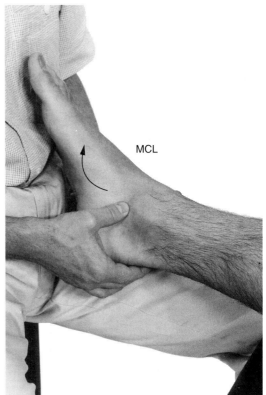

Fig. 6.42

calcaneus through to the musculotendinous junction with the gastrocnemius and soleus muscles (Figure 6.43) (*). The tendon is very thick and fibrous in nature, designed to transfer very high loads during various forms of gait.

ii) Also palpate the lateral and medial edge of the AT at the calcaneal insertion and as the common tendon blends at the musculotendinous junction of the gastrocnemius–soleus muscles (Figure 6.44) (*). Ask the patient to plantar flex the foot against resistance in order to appreciate the tendon under mechanical load.

iii) Palpate the bellies of the soleus (S), gastrocnemius (G) and the musculotendinous junction (MTJ) during this palpation exercise (Figure 6.45). These are highly influential structures in the gait mechanism and rear foot biomechanics. *Ask the patient to resist against plantar flexion in order to appreciate the power in this muscle complex but also to differentiate the two components morphologically. The patient's leg is flexed at the knee to isolate the soleus primarily during the resisted manual test.*

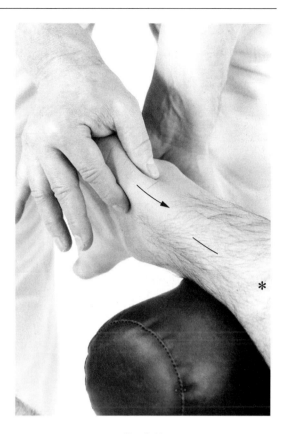

Fig. 6.43

VASCULAR STRUCTURES OF THE LOWER EXTREMITY

Assessing arterial pulses is a standard examination procedure for a patient presenting with back and leg pain. This constitutes triage procedures common during physical examination in order to differentiate the aetiology. This is also important for appropriate referral considerations.

Establishing bilaterally equal and patent arterial supply to the lower extremities is an important screening procedure of the physical examination. Ruling out vascular claudication is vitally important when establishing a differential diagnosis for a patient presenting with leg and/or foot pain.

Therefore, locating important arterial structures of the lower limb represents basic examination procedures for the undergraduate.

This section will present how to locate three major arteries of the lower extremity.

Dorsalis pedis artery (DP)

i) Support the foot as described in Figure 6.3. Use the 1st and 2nd finger pads to locate the artery, *not the thumb pad*. The artery is normally located between the extensor hallucis longus and extensor digitorum longus tendons at the midfoot region (Figure 6.46) (*). Though the

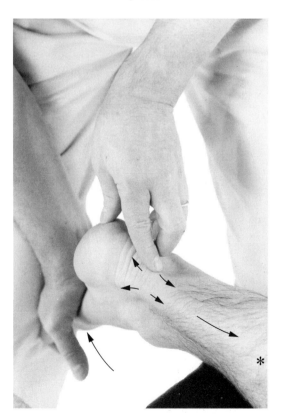

Fig. 6.44

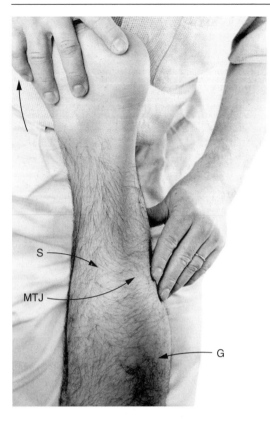

Fig. 6.45

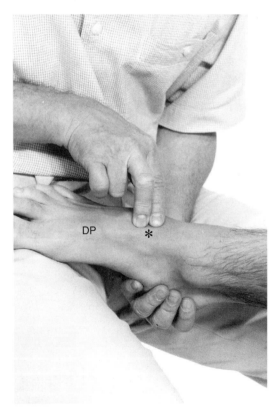

Fig. 6.46

artery is superficial it can be difficult to find and is reported to be absent 15% of the time in the general population. Its anatomical location can vary considerably between individuals.

ii) If difficulties are encountered establishing the location of the artery, then lightly grasp the dorsum of the foot and generally feel and appreciate the arterial pulse of the foot or have the patient dorsiflex the great toe to identify the EHL and EDL tendons to assist in finding the arterial pulse (Figure 6.47).

Posterior tibial artery (PT)

i) Support the foot as described in Figure 6.3 placing the foot in a neutral relaxed position. The artery is located on the medial aspect of the lower extremity proximal to the posterior aspect of the medial malleolus (MM) between the flexor hallucis longus and flexor digitorum longus tendons (*). Use the 1st and 2nd fingers to palpate for the arterial pulse (Figure 6.48).

Popliteal artery (PA)

i) The PA is located very deep within the popliteal space in the posterior knee region. Place the patient prone and flex the knee to approximately 45 degrees to relax the popliteal structures. Using the 1st and 2nd finger pads probe the posterior knee region to locate the popliteal artery which lies close to the posterior knee capsule (Figure 6.49).

FUNDAMENTAL JOINT PLAY SKILLS OF THE FOOT/ANKLE COMPLEX

Developing the ability to appreciate the subtle natural spring and compliance associated with the synovial joints of the foot/ankle is a necessary pre-manipulative skill. Though the foot has a wide range of global motion in various complex axes and planes, it is the passive joint play of the individual articulations that collectively contributes to this overall function. The foot/ankle complex functions both in weight bearing and gait propulsion requiring both stability and flexibility from the various regions of the foot/ankle. Optimal function of all the articulations of the foot/ankle complex are required for appropriate weight transfer and energy conservation.

Learning to appreciate subtle passive involuntary motion of the major articulations of the foot/ankle is a prerequisite for assessment and manipulative inter-

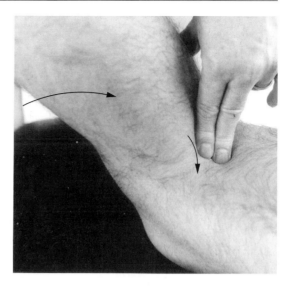

Fig. 6.49

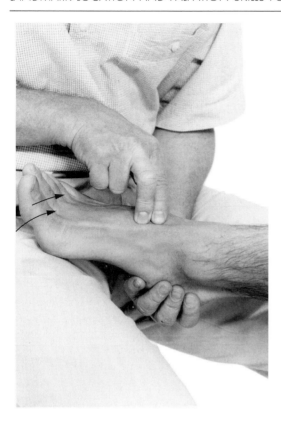

Fig. 6.47

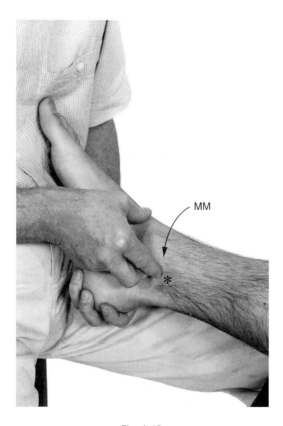

Fig. 6.48

vention. These skills are similar to those presented in the previous chapters and constitute basic psycho-motor acquisition and joint analysis procedures. At this point in undergraduate training applying new anatomical landmark location and palpation skills requires clinical application and frameworking.

This section presents an overview of joint play skills for the foot/ankle complex. Emphasis is placed upon reasonable anatomical accuracy, joint location, posture and joint play challenge motor skills. Importance will be placed upon introducing an appropriate amount of force across or along the respective joints to engage the natural spring or compliance that is an inherent feature of all synovial joints. Factors such as joint architecture, surrounding holding elements and axes of motion will all influence joint play magnitudes and performance. The average joint play of a synovial joint has been estimated to be somewhere in the range of 3–5 mm (Mennell, 1964; Mennell, 1990; Mennell, 1991). This is a reasonable reference point to begin assimilating these motor skills and appreciation.

Talocrural joint (tibiotalar) – anterior-posterior and posterior-anterior glide

i) Grasp the distal tibia and fibula just proximal to the medial malleolus with the web of cephalad hand (Figure 6.50) (*). The other hand grasps the dome of the talus with the web of the hand and the index and middle fingers reach around and support the posterior aspect of the talus and the calcaneus respec-

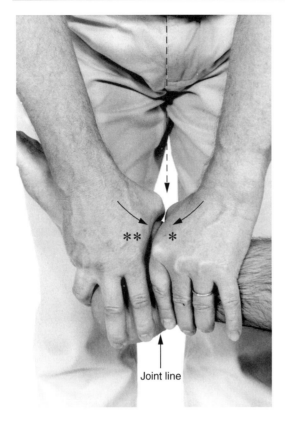

Fig. 6.50

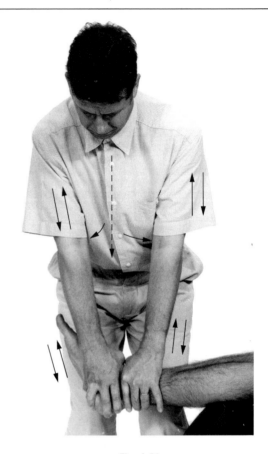

Fig. 6.51

tively (**). The hands should be positioned very close in order to isolate and stabilize the ankle joint proper.

ii) Maintain the mortice joint in a neutral position with the joint slightly dorsiflexed and using both hand contacts apply a simultaneous translational force in opposite directions, anterior to posterior and posterior to anterior through both hands isolating the joint play movement of the mortice joint (Figure 6.51). The movement should be generated through the shoulders and upper chest wall with the elbows and wrist remaining firm to guide the joint play force across the joint.

Talocrural joint (tibiotalar) – long axis distraction

i) Sit with the patient's leg over the lap of the practitioner with the leg flexed at the hip and knee. Place the web of one hand over the dome of the talus and the other over the superior aspect of the calcaneus. Both thumbs should meet just inferior to the medial malleolus (Figure 6.52) (*).

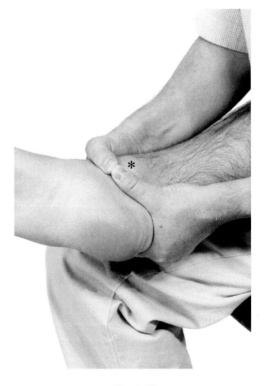

Fig. 6.52

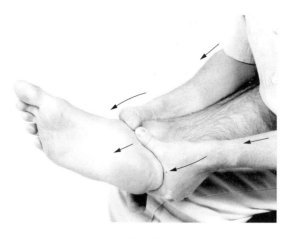

Fig. 6.53

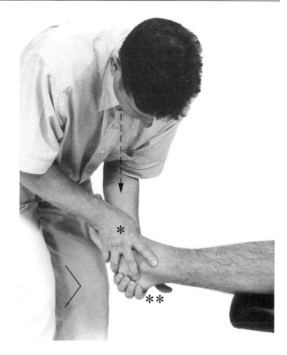

Fig. 6.54

ii) Stabilize the knee and hip and maintain the foot in a neutral position. Simultaneously apply a distraction force with both hands assessing the joint play movement of the mortice joint (Figure 6.53). Joint play force should be generated through the shoulder and anterior chest wall in order to overcome the tissue resistance at the joint level.

Subtalar joint – eversion and inversion

i) Wrap the middle finger of the caudad hand around the cuboid and the index finger and thumb (Figure 6.54) (*) round the talus and grasp the calcaneus in the palm of the cephalad hand (**). Note the low ski or fencer stance with the sternal notch over the joint complex to improve overall efficiency.

ii) Stabilize the forefoot with the caudad hand (S) and move the calcaneus medially and laterally introducing inversion and eversion joint play springing movement at the subtalar joint (Figure 6.55). Movements should be oscillatory and repetitive in nature to assess the subtalar joint play. Maintain sternal notch position posture so all the movement is taking place as a result of small levers through the calcaneal contact.

Metatarsophalangeal joint (MTP) – anterior-posterior and long axis distraction

i) Stabilize the head of the first MTP with the 1ˢᵗ finger and thumb of the left hand wrapped around in a clasp-like fashion (Figure 6.56) (*). The other hand contacts the proximal

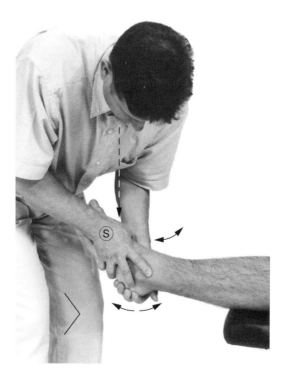

Fig. 6.55

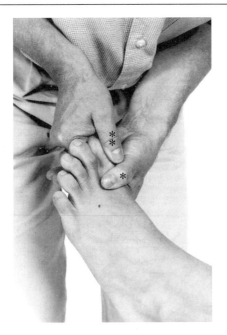

Fig. 6.56

end of the first phalanx close to the joint space using a thumb and 1st finger contact (**).

ii)   Keep the cephalad (left) hand contact firm and stable (S). Move the proximal phalanx contact in an up and down fashion assessing the anterior to posterior and posterior to anterior joint play. Also assess long axis distraction by applying distraction force along the axis of the 1st

metatarsal (Figure 6.57). *This procedure can be used for all the MTP joints.*

Intermetatarsals – anterior-posterior and posterior-anterior glide

i)   Grasp the first and second metatarsals with 1st and 2nd fingers and thumb in a clasp-like fashion. The foot should be overhanging the table with the foot/ankle in a neutral position. Move both contacts together in opposite directions to introduce a shear joint play springing movement between tarsals. *This joint play procedure can be utilized for all intertarsal combinations.*

General foot joint play scan skills

i)   Cup the calcaneus with one hand and wrap the other hand over the dorsum of the foot. The thumb of the cephalad hand projects forward in order to palpate the structures of the foot from the medial and lateral plantar aspect. Systematically beginning from the cuboid, plantar flex (PF) the mid/forefoot over the contact thumb to assess the individual joint play spring of the individual osseous structures of the foot to include the lateral and medial joint structures including the cuboid, navicular, first cuneiform and 1st metatarsal (Figure 6.58).

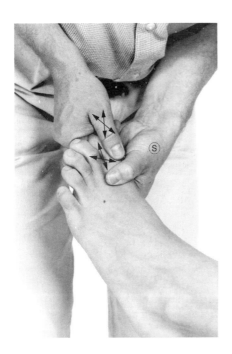

Fig. 6.57

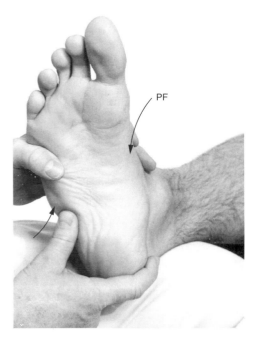

Fig. 6.58

Section 2 The knee

This section will cover the knee complex

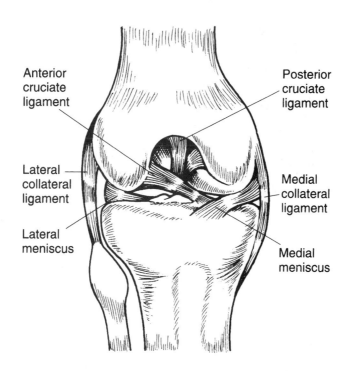

Anterior cruciate ligament

Posterior cruciate ligament

Lateral collateral ligament

Medial collateral ligament

Lateral meniscus

Medial meniscus

ACTIVE RANGE OF MOTION AND LANDMARK LOCATION

i) A general appreciation of overall knee joint range of motion should be assessed prior to palpation and landmark location. Place the patient prone and move the heel towards the buttock fully. This represents 130–140 degrees of knee flexion (Figure 6.59). The knee is capable of 180 degrees of extension from full flexion.

ii) Position the patient in the supine posture with the hip and knee flexed to 90 degrees of flexion. Grasp the knee joint midline with the thumb and 1st finger and use the heel to rotate the tibia on the femur, approximately 5 degrees of both internal (Figure 6.60a) and external rotation (Figure 6.60b) of the tibiofemoral joint. This represents important passive joint play of the patellofemoral joint complex.

iii) The optimal palpation position for locating and examining most knee structures is with the patient in the supine position with the knee flexed to approximately 90 degrees with the foot flat and the practitioner sitting over the lateral aspect of the patient's foot to stabilize the leg and knee (*) (Figure 6.61).

iv) The optimal hand posture for palpation of the knee and related structures is wrapping both hands around the knee freeing both thumbs and fingers to probe and locate various anatomical landmarks both on the anterior and posterior surfaces. The fingers wrap around the

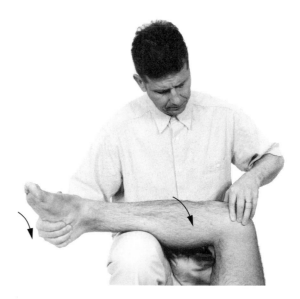

Fig. 6.60a

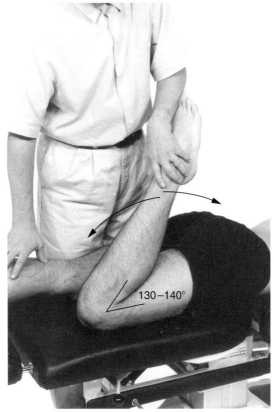

Fig. 6.59

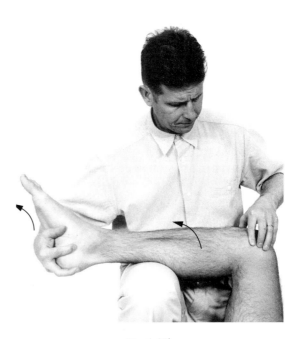

Fig. 6.60b

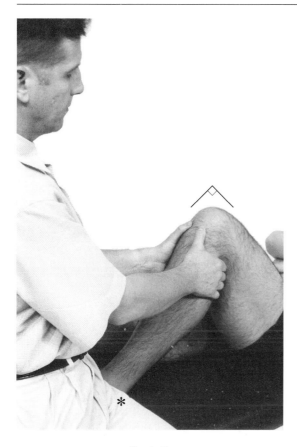

Fig. 6.61

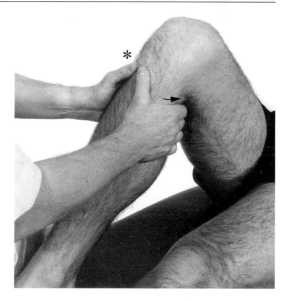

Fig. 6.62

popliteal space and the thumbs will naturally fall on the region on each side of the patellar tendon over the medial and lateral aspect of the knee joint line (*) (Figure 6.62).

OSSEOUS LANDMARKS

Medial aspect of the knee

Tibial tubercle and patellar tendon

i)   Place the patient in the position described in Figure 6.61. Follow the patellar (infrapatellar) tendon down or the tibial crest up to the outgrowth of bone, the tibial tubercle (Figure 6.63a) (*). It is the attachment point for the patellar tendon, which has important patellofemoral function. The thumbs or 1st and 2nd fingers can be used to palpate this common landmark of the knee structure (Figure 6.63b).

ii) Move the thumbs superiorly to locate and palpate the patellar tendon as it attaches to the tibial tubercle and the inferior aspect of the

pole of the patella (Figure 6.64). This structure is a thick band-like structure that has significant clinical implications in knee injuries.

Medial tibial plateau and tibial condyle

i)   Move the thumb up and medially from the tibial tubercle to appreciate the depression and flare of the tibial plateau (Figure 6.65) (*). Continue towards the joint line and probe the non-articulating aspect of the tibial condyle.

ii) Continue to move the palpating thumb superiorly to find and palpate the tibial plateau and the medial knee joint line (Figure 6.66) (*). Moving the thumb laterally at this point will appreciate more of the medial joint line and the closer the articulation with the femur.

Medial femoral condyle

i)   Move the thumb further superior across the joint line and medial to the patella to locate and probe the medial femoral condyle. The condyle is the articulating surface and is relatively smooth in relation to the patella (Figure 6.67).

ii) Continue to move the palpating thumb medially to find the edge of the medial femoral condyle, which can be palpated distally through to the joint line (Figure 6.68).

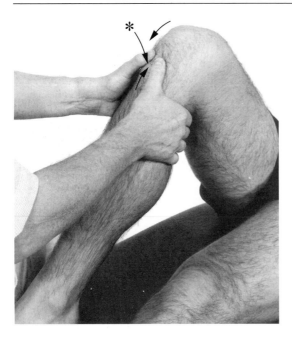

Fig. 6.63a

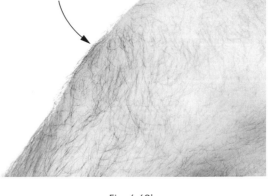

Fig. 6.63b

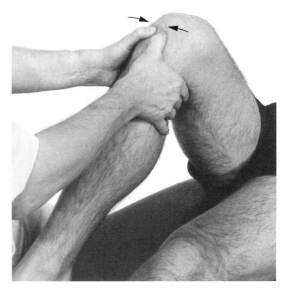

Fig. 6.64

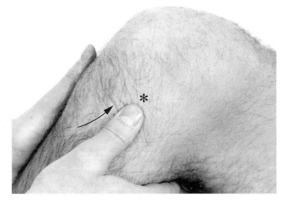

Fig. 6.65

Adductor tubercle and medial epicondyle

i) Move back to the medial femoral condyle and the edge of the condyle. Continue to palpate posteriorly from this point until one encounters an osseous elevation found at the lower edge of the vastus medialis (VM), the medial femoral condyle (Figure 6.69) (*).

ii) The adductor tubercle serves as an attachment point for the adductor magnus and is essentially an osseous thickening of the larger medial epicondyle (Figure 6.70) (*) which is found by palpating posterior to the medial epicondyle.

iii) At this point the large knee muscles are visible and palpable including the vastus medialis (VM) and the adductor group (AG) (Figure 6.71). These muscles are important stabilizing components of the knee and are crucial to address during any knee rehabilitation programme.

Patella

i) Assume the basic palpation hand position as depicted in Figure 6.61. Use both thumbs to define the outline of the patella from the superior to inferior poles including the medial and lateral borders (Figure 6.72). The patella

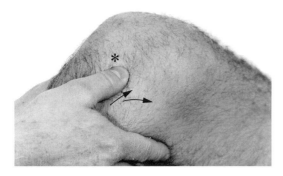

Fig. 6.66

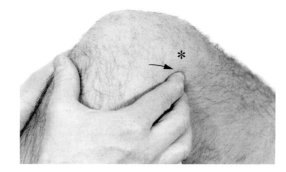

Fig. 6.70

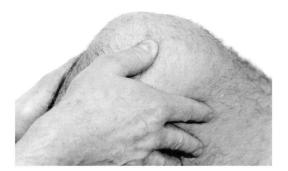

Fig. 6.67

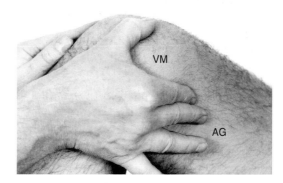

Fig. 6.71

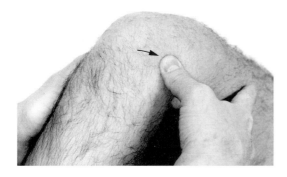

Fig. 6.68

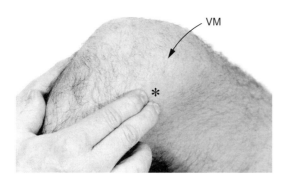

Fig. 6.69

has important clinical significance as a site of muscle attachment and an important component of overall knee function.

Lateral aspect of the knee

Lateral tibial plateau

i)   Place the patient in standard palpating posture as in Figure 6.61 exposing the lateral aspect of the knee for palpation and anatomical landmark location exercise (Figure 6.73). The clinician should sit against the lateral edge of the patient's foot straddling the table in order to stabilize the knee.

ii) Locate the soft tissue depression just lateral to the patellar tendon. Palpate deep into this region to feel the edge of the lateral tibial plateau. Palpate along its edge to the point where you feel the junction of the tibia and femur at the lateral joint line (Figure 6.74) (*).

iii) Continue to palpate along the tibial plateau and more laterally along the lateral tibiofemoral joint line (Figure 6.75).

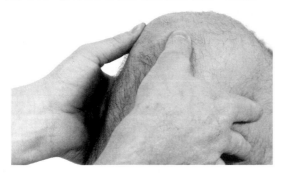

Fig. 6.72

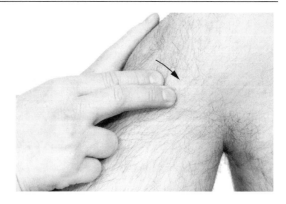

Fig. 6.75

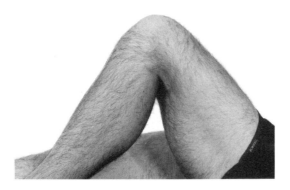

Fig. 6.73

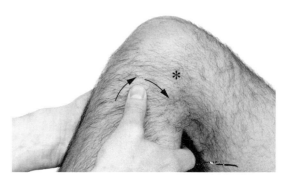

Fig. 6.76

Lateral tibial tubercle

i) Just below the lateral tibial plateau is the large prominence of bone called the lateral tibial tubercle. This is located just lateral to the patellar tendon and the tibial tubercle (Figure 6.76) (*).

Lateral femoral condyle

i) Palpate laterally and superiorly from the lateral joint line to locate the lateral femoral condyle

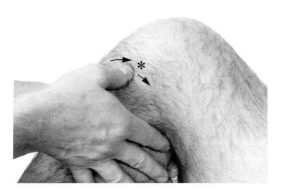

Fig. 6.74

and the sharp edge of the lateral femoral condyle (Figure 6.77a) (*). Maintain the joint line of the tibia and femur in perspective during palpation. Using the 1st and 2nd digit finger pads palpate the sharpness of the lateral femoral condyle (Figure 6.77b) (*).

Lateral femoral epicondyle

i) Continue to palpate laterally and locate the bony lateral femoral epicondyle which lies laterally to the lateral femoral condyle (Figure 6.78).

Head of the fibula

i) Palpate inferior from the lateral femoral condyle to locate the head of the fibula (Figure 6.79). The fibular head is located at the same level as the tibial tubercle (*). This provides an excellent landmark to locate another. Use the 1st and 2nd finger pads to delineate the fibular head morphology.

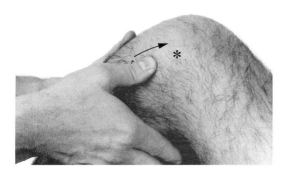

Fig. 6.77a

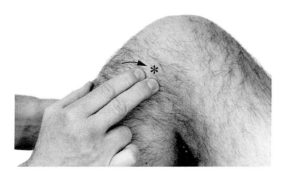

Fig. 6.77b

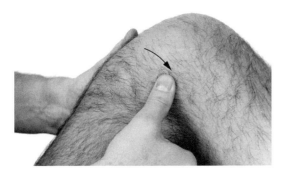

Fig. 6.78

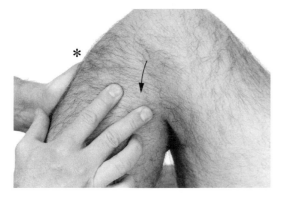

Fig. 6.79

Trochlear groove (TG)

i) The TG is the depression located between the medial and lateral femoral condyles where the patella sits and glides during various movements including gait (Figure 6.80) (*). This region has clinical importance relative to patellofemoral syndrome and patellar pathomechanics.

ii) With the thumb and 1st finger pad the medial and lateral walls of the TG can be palpated (Figure 6.81). The lateral wall is higher than the medial and has clinical significance (*). Note the soft tissues of the region.

Inferior surface of the patella

i) With the leg extended and relaxed in contact with the table, move the patella medially and with the palpating 1st digit palpate the inferior medial surface of the patella at its border (Figure 6.82) (*). This region has clinical significance in patellofemoral syndromes.

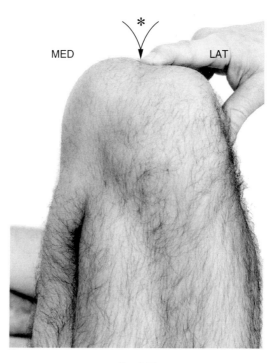

Fig. 6.80

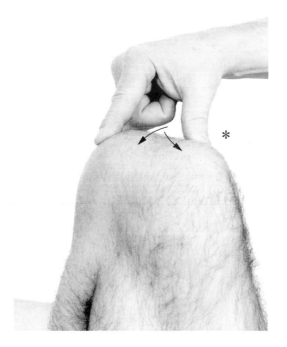

Fig. 6.81

SOFT TISSUE LANDMARKS – MUSCULAR STRUCTURES

Quadriceps

i)   With the patient lying supine identify the various quadriceps components including the vastus lateralis (VL), rectus femoris (RF) and vastus medialis (VM) (Figure 6.83).

ii) Palpate the muscular structures individually to appreciate their delineation and position as part of the patellofemoral complex (Figure 6.84).

Biceps femoris

i)   With the patient in the supine posture palpate the tendon of the biceps femoris just prior to its insertion into the lateral condyle of the tibia below the knee joint line (Figure 6.85).

Iliotibial band

i)   Palpate superiorly and anterior to the biceps femoris tendon to assess the iliotibial band which is a large fibrous band located on the

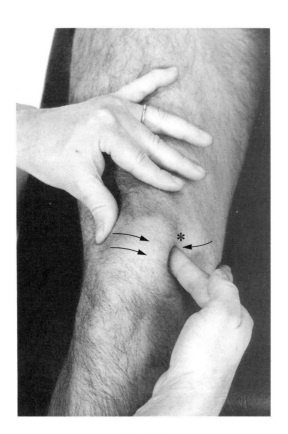

Fig. 6.82

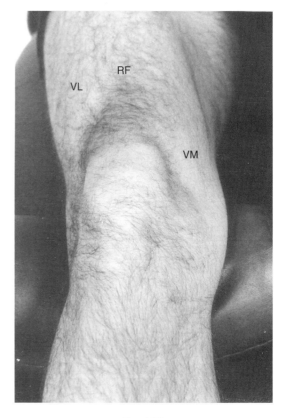

Fig. 6.83

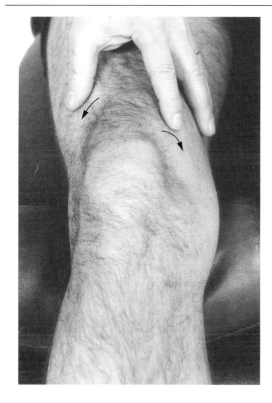

Fig. 6.84

lateral aspect of the thigh overlying the vastus lateralis inserting into the femoral and tibial condyles assisting in stabilizing the lateral aspect of the knee (Figure 6.86). This structure has significant clinical implications particularly in runners.

Medial and lateral head of gastrocnemius

i) With the patient lying in the prone position flex the knee to relax the posterior muscular structures. The medial head is found by palpating just below the popliteal space. The medial head is large and inserts into the femur above the knee joint line (Figure 6.87).

ii) Palpate laterally to delineate the lateral head of the gastrocnemius (Figure 6.88). The lateral

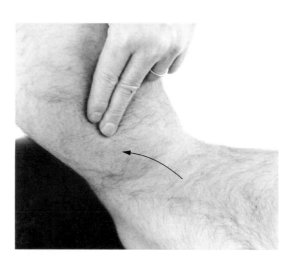

Fig. 6.87

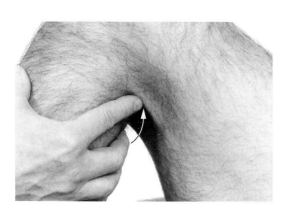

Fig. 6.85

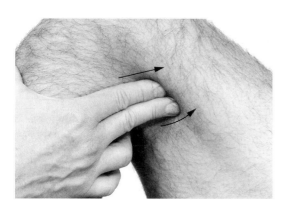

Fig. 6.86

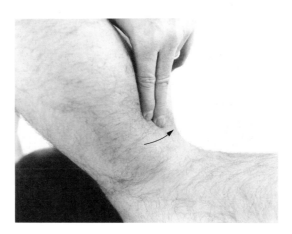

Fig. 6.88

head is also a large muscle mass that inserts above the knee joint line.

Semitendinosus (ST), gracilis (G), sartorius (S), pes anserine bursa (PA)

i) With the patient lying prone, observe and palpate the muscular structures that pass the medial knee joint line including sartorius (S), gracilis (G) and semitendinosus (ST). This group of muscles inserts at a common point just below the tibial plateau medial to the tibial tubercle on the tibia (Figure 6.89)(*). At this common insertion lies the pes anserine bursa which has clinical significance for many active patients.

SOFT TISSUE LANDMARKS – LIGAMENTOUS STRUCTURES

Lateral collateral ligament (LCL)

i) Place the patient supine and simultaneously flex the hip and knee and externally rotate the leg by placing the heel of the left leg

over the suprapatellar region of the opposite leg (Figure 6.90) (*). The knee should be flexed to 90 degrees. This helps to relax the iliotibial band making palpation of the ligament more accessible.

ii) Palpate along the lateral joint line to find and palpate the thick LCL. The ligament is located more posterior on the lateral aspect of the knee (Figure 6.91) (*). The ligament joins the femur and tibia and has clinical significance as a result of repetitive strain injuries and contact sports trauma.

Medial collateral ligament (MCL)

i) In order to locate the MCL find the medial joint line and move posterior to palpate the ligament which is broad in nature and part of the joint capsule. Palpate across the fibres

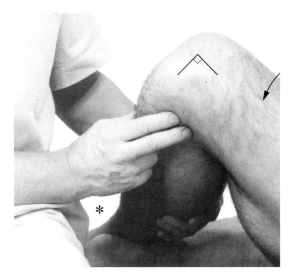

Fig. 6.90

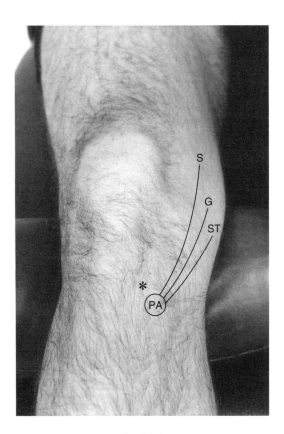

Fig. 6.89

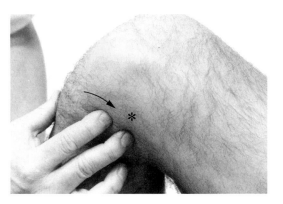

Fig. 6.91

and palpate cephalad to palpate the ligament as it attaches to the medial epicondyle of the femur (Figure 6.92). This ligament is best palpated with the knee slightly flexed. This ligament also has clinical significance in repetitive strain injuries and contact sport trauma and is usually related to the medial meniscus and anterior cruciate during more serious injuries.

Medial (MM) and lateral meniscus (LM)

i) The MM and LM are best palpated with the knee in slight flexion as both menisci disappear on full extension. The LM is found by probing the lateral joint space along the lateral tibial plateau (*). The thumb or finger pads can be employed to assist this exercise (Figure 6.93). The LM is attached to the popliteus muscle and not to the LCL which has significant clinical importance in chronic knee injuries. The MM is found in the same fashion as the LM deep along the medial joint line (**). The MM is best found with the tibia internally rotated. Clinically, tears are more common in the MM.

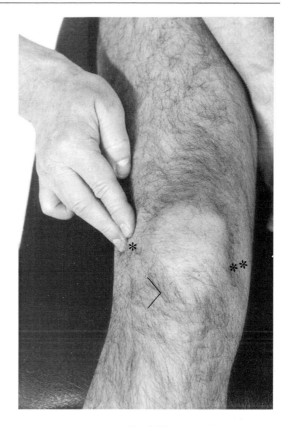

Fig. 6.93

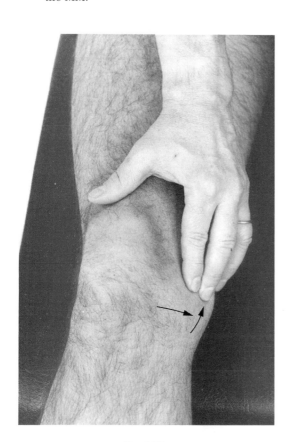

Fig. 6.92

FUNDAMENTAL JOINT PLAY SKILLS OF THE PATELLOFEMORAL COMPLEX

As with the foot/ankle the same rationale regarding joint play assessment and fundamental skills will be presented as a basic overview of a very complex joint structure. This exercise will utilize aspects of newly learned palpation and landmark location skills and place them into a clinical assessment context. It is important to visualize the anatomical components during both palpation and joint play assessment in order to enhance newly acquired skills. Additional reading and references will be included at the end of the chapter.

Tibiofemoral joint (TFJ) – anterior-posterior (A-P) and posterior-anterior (P-A) glide

i) Place the patient in the supine posture with the knee to be assessed flexed to 90 degrees. Lightly but firmly wrap the hands around the entire knee joint and sit on the lateral aspect of the patient's foot to stabilize the leg and knee during examination. The thumbs, web of the hand and the fingers should be positioned below the joint line in contact with the tibia only (Figure 6.94) (*) and the practitioner's arms should be tucked into the side of the body (**). Assess the subtle joint compliance by applying a short, quick movement along the joint line, initially P-A and then A-P, appreciating the natural spring and give to this joint. This joint play force is generated through the practitioner's shoulders and anterior chest wall musculature in a coordinated movement. These movements are required for normal joint mechanics and function and have clinical significance. Don't be aggressive when learning to appreciate these subtle joint movements.

Tibiofibular joint – anterior-posterior and posterior-anterior glide

i)   Adopt a similar posture to that described in Figure 6.94 both to palpate and stabilize the patient. Lightly but firmly wrap the thumb and index finger around the head of the fibula in a clasp-like fashion (Figure 6.95) (*). Assess the subtle TFJ play by first moving the fibula from P-A and then A-P in a short quick movement generated by the shoulder and anterior chest wall musculature as shown in Figure 6.95 (**). These subtle movements have clinical significance particularly in chronic knee pain presentation.

Patellofemoral joint – superior-inferior, inferior-superior, medial-lateral, lateral-medial glide

i)   Position the patient in the supine posture with the knee relaxed and fully extended. This posture isolates patellar movement and stabilizes the tibiofemoral joint. Place the thumb and index finger pads of both hands at the superior and inferior pole of the patella (Figure 6.96).

ii) Move the patella from inferior to superior along the femoral condyle appreciating the easy glide and play of the patella using a bilateral finger-thumb contact (Figure 6.97). Both contacts should move in unison.

iii) Move the patella superior to inferior along the same track using the same contact and movement pattern (Figure 6.98).

iv) Place both thumbs over the lateral border of the patella with the hands in an arched posture. Move the thumbs medially in unison with some slight ulnar deviation to assist the lateral-medial glide of the patella (Figure 6.99). There should be quite a bit of movement observed as with superior-inferior and inferior-superior play.

v)   Place the index finger pads along the medial border of the patella with the hands still in an arched and slightly ulnar deviated posture (Figure 6.100) (*). Move the fingers together against the medial patella border to introduce medial-lateral play.

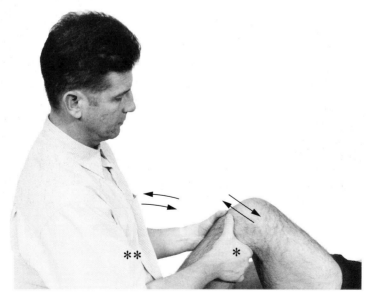

Fig. 6.94

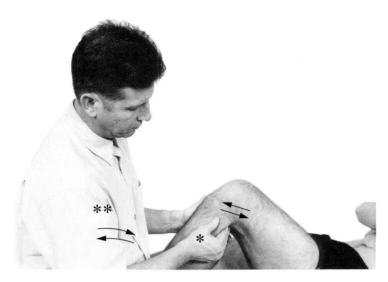

Fig. 6.95

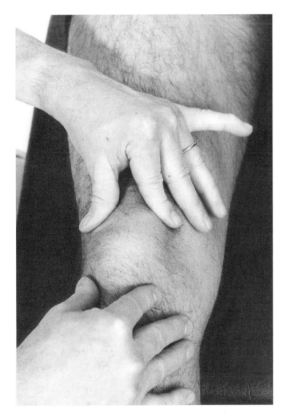

Fig. 6.96

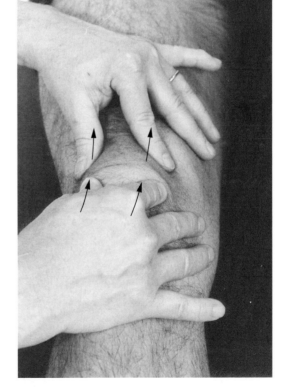

Fig. 6.97

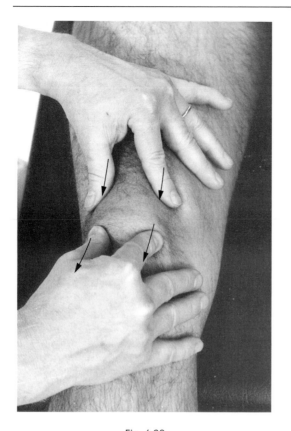

Fig. 6.98

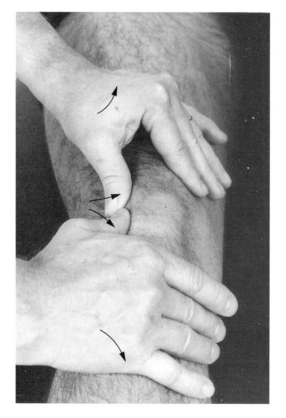

Fig. 6.99

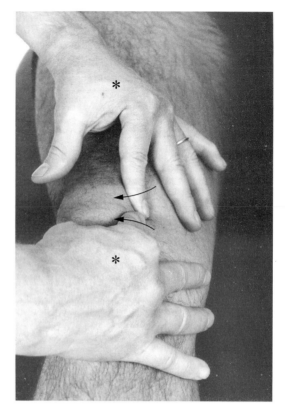

Fig. 6.100

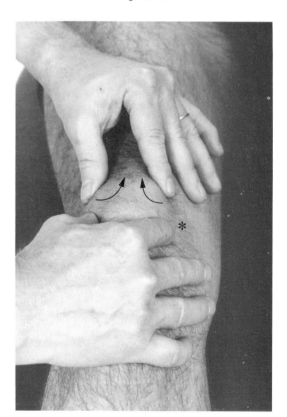

Fig. 6.101

vi) Place the thumb and index fingers as shown in Figure 6.96 but tuck the digit pads under the inferior edge of the patella at both poles (Figure 6.101) (*). Grasp the patella and slightly lift the patella away from the femoral condyle to assess the axial lift and give of the patella. This movement has clinical significance with respect to chronic knee pain presentation.

Section 3 The hip joint

This section will cover the hip complex

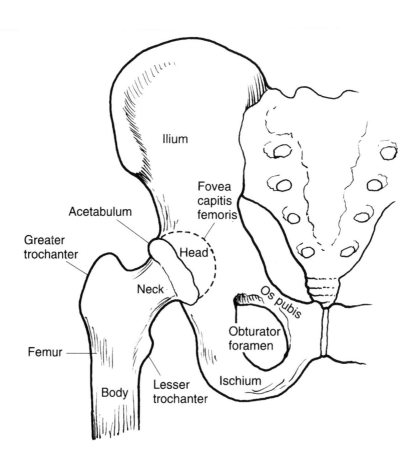

INTRODUCTION

The hip joint is considered the most stable joint in the body and, as a result, various joint structures are inaccessible for direct palpation by the practitioner. The hip joint represents an important component of the pelvic ring and warrants investigation when assessing patients presenting with various forms of back pain. There are a few important osseous and soft tissue landmarks of note with respect to the hip joint which require identification. There are also a few joint play skills that assess fundamental joint play analysis of the hip joint to appreciate its complexity as well as its stability.

LANDMARK LOCATION

Osseous landmark location

Greater trochanter (GT)

i) Place the patient in the side lying posture and palpate down or inferior from the pelvic crest over the lateral aspect of the thigh. The GT is the only osseous structure located in this region (Figure. 6.102) (*). The GT is an attachment point for a number of important pelvic muscles, particularly the external rotators and abductors of the hip.

Ischial tuberosity (IT)

i) The IT is located at the level of the gluteal fold approximately in the middle of the buttock. The IT can be found by palpating medially

from the GT or inferiorly from the PSIS (Figure 6.103). The large gluteus maximus overlies this osseous structure (*).

Anterior superior iliac spine (ASIS)

i) Place the patient in the supine position. The bony ASIS is visible in most people but is located lateral to the umbilicus and slightly inferior (Figure 6.104). The ASIS serves as an attachment point for muscle and ligament and is regarded as an important pelvic landmark (*).

Soft tissue landmark location

Inguinal ligament (IL)

i) Palpate the IL just medial and inferior to the ASIS (Figure 6.105). The IL extends medially to the pubic tubercles. The IL has clinical significance in chronic back pain and may be a source of recurrent pain.

Gluteus medius (GM)

i) Place the patient in the side lying posture. Ask the patient actively to abduct the leg and observe the bulk of the GM (Figure 6.106) (*).

ii) Palpate this muscle complex, both in a contracted and non-contracted state to appreciate the anterior (Figure 6.107) (*) and posterior fibres (**). These structures have clinical significance.

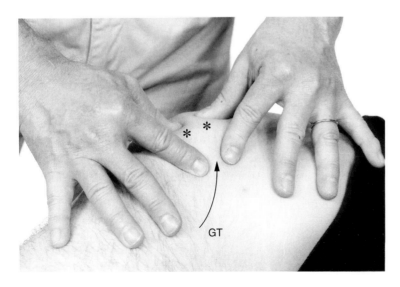

Fig. 6.102

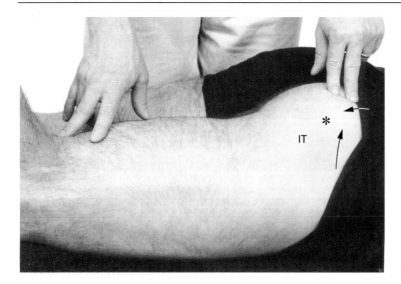

Fig. 6.103

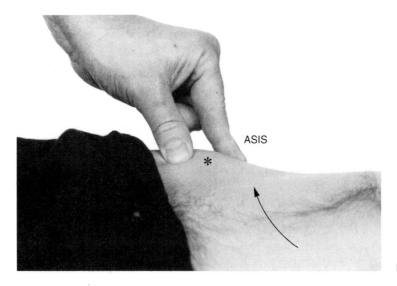

Fig. 6.104

JOINT PLAY SKILLS AND RANGE OF MOTION

Figure 4 (flexion, abduction, external rotation)

i) Place the patient in the supine posture. Flex the right knee and place the foot over the supra-patellar region of the left leg (Figure 6.108) (*). This places the right hip in the Figure 4 or flexed, abducted and externally rotated provocation position. This position also defines the amount of rotation at the hip joint and is a standard orthopaedic test for hip stability.

There is a great deal of variation within the normal population with respect to range of motion of the hip joint considering all planes of motion. In order to assess the joint play of the hip in this position stabilize the opposite hip with the cephalad hand over the ASIS(s) and gently and progressively push the knee down towards the table to evaluate the passive movement and elastic elements of the hip joint (Figure 6.108). Introduce repetitive oscillations at this point to appreciate fully the elastic barrier and condition of the joint stabilizing structures. Ensure that the sternal notch (*) is located over the hip joint being assessed to maintain postural stability and efficiency during the performance of this examination pro-

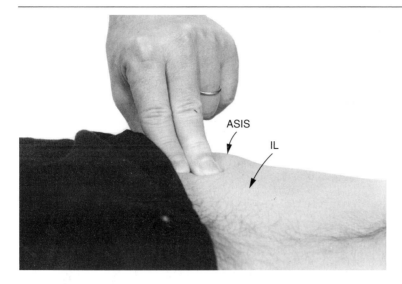

Fig. 6.105

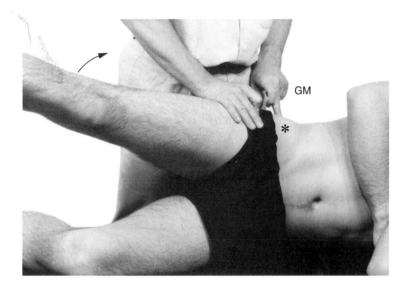

Fig. 6.106

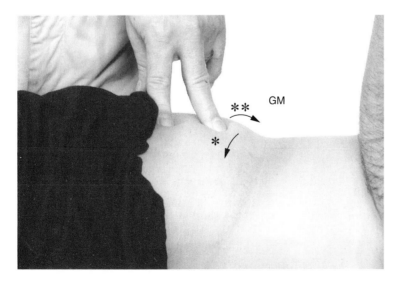

Fig. 6.107

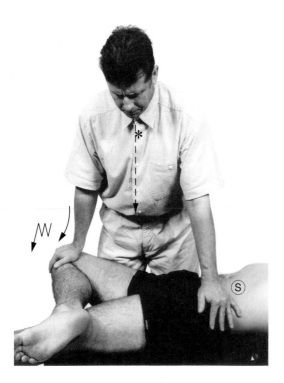

Fig. 6.108

cedure. Stand on the ipsilateral side being examined. This particular test has clinical significance as a hip provocation test for hip pathology. The *femoral triangle* can be assessed in this position including the *femoral artery*, which is an important vascular structure in the assessment of the lower extremity.

Internal rotation (IR) – (supine)

i) With the patient in the supine posture position the right knee and hip at 90 degrees. Place the cephalad hand over the lateral aspect of the knee and the caudad hand grasps the medial side of the rear foot. Externally rotate the tibia to introduce internal rotation of the femur and hip joint. Appreciate the passive elastic feel of the joint near the end range of motion at which point repetitive oscillations are introduced to evaluate the state of the elastic barrier of the hip joint in internal rotation (Figure 6.109). Ensure that the sternal notch is located over or close to the joint being assessed. Keep the arms close to the body to control lever action across the joint (*).

External rotation (ER) – (supine)

i) With the patient in the same posture, reverse the hand positions and assess ET of the hip joint. Maintain the hip and knee at 90 degrees. Place the cephalad hand on the medial knee and the caudad hand over the lateral aspect of the ankle/foot region and simultaneously internally rotate the tibia producing external rotation of the hip. At the point of full ET assess the elastic barrier of the joint by applying repetitive oscillations in order to challenge the passive elastic elements of the hip in ET (Figure 6.110).

Posterior shear (PS)

i) Place the patient in the supine position with the hip at 90 degrees (Figure 6.111) (*). Position the hands over the knee in an interlocked overlapped position (**). Ensure that the sternal notch is directly over the hand position. Plantar flex the rear foot and bring the body weight over the knee contact and apply downward compression to assess the elastic properties of the posterior hip capsule. Ensure that the practitioner's hands and chest wall are in contact to reduce overall leverage.

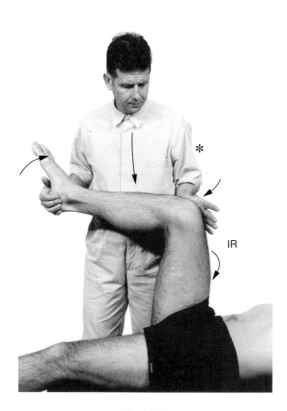

Fig. 6.109

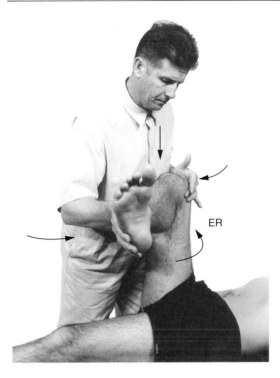

Fig. 6.110

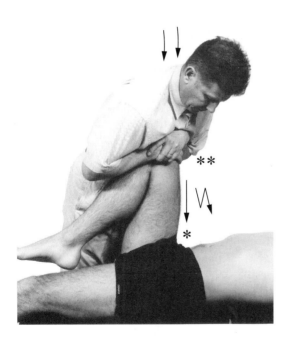

Fig. 6.111

SUMMARY

This chapter has presented basic osseous and soft tissue landmark location instruction plus rudimentary joint play evaluation of the foot/ankle, knee and hip joints. These are fundamental skills for the manual therapist to acquire prior to introduction of manipulative skills of the spine, pelvis and extremity joints.

REFERENCES

Mennell, J.M. (1964) Preamble. In: *Joint Pain: Diagnosis and Treatment Using Manipulative Techniques* (Mennell, J.M. ed.). pp. 1–11. Little Brown & Company, Boston.

Mennell, J.M. (1990) Another critical look at the diagnosis "joint dysfunction" in synovial joints of the cervical spine. *J Manipulative Physiol Ther.* **13**, 7–12.

Mennell, J.M. (1991) The manipulable lesion: joint play, joint dysfunction and joint manipulation. In: *Functional Soft Tissue Examination and Treatment by Manual Methods* (Hammer, W. ed.). pp. 191–196. Aspen Publishers, Gaithersburg.

FURTHER READING

Bergmann, T., Peterson, D., Lawrence, D. (1993) *Chiropractic Technique.* Churchill Livingstone, London.

Byfield, D. (1996) *Chiropractic Manipulative Skills.* Butterworth-Heinemann, Oxford.

Magee, D. (1987) *Orthopaedic Physical Assessment.* W.B. Saunders Company, London.

7

Basic palpation and anatomical landmark identification skills for the upper extremity

Stuart Kinsinger

INTRODUCTION

Palpation of the upper extremity with reference to specific anatomical landmarks and soft tissue configurations is a learned skill requiring many hours of practice and concentration. This is also a very important region from a clinical perspective, particularly in many sports-related injuries. Therefore, a strong basic anatomical knowledge must be established prior to embarking upon learning these psychomotor skill sets with any degree of proficiency. It has also been reported that visual and mental imagery may enhance complex psychomotor skill learning. Following appreciation of various structural markers, the next step is to introduce standard palpation protocols to analyse the static and dynamic qualities of the articulations of the upper extremity. Lack of articular movement has been identified as a principal chiropractic tenet and a fundamental requirement prior to manipulative intervention. This analysis is underpinned by a descriptive theory outlining the active and passive range of motion of diarthroidial joints. It also classifies which particular holding elements (capsular and ligamentous) are challenged during each specific palpation procedure, permitting the clinician to establish a reasonably accurate diagnosis of dysfunction. The procedure should identify which aspect of the joint range of motion is impaired (active, passive, joint play).

This chapter will focus on landmark identification and passive joint play assessment. These are rudimentary joint analysis techniques and play an important role in establishing a clinical diagnosis in chiropractic practice. Joint play is described as the natural compliance of a joint in its neutral or end range position.

This chapter will also focus on appropriate postural skills for the practitioner when learning and performing these basic palpatory skills for the upper extremity. This chapter will also present a variety of soft tissue palpation techniques plus identification of a number of important anatomical landmarks in the upper extremity. Learning an efficient posture during this initializing period will provide the framework for more complex psychomotor skills implemented later during undergraduate education.

Injuries to the articulations of the upper extremity are common. It is therefore important for the undergraduate to develop a working knowledge of the functional anatomy and joint mechanics of all major extremity articulations in order to provide management and care for these clinical conditions. Furthermore, the shoulder girdle is a very complex multijoint structure that is subject to overuse and asymmetrical mechanical loading during the performance of a number of common activities. This places additional stress on the associated soft tissue and ligamentous holding elements contributing to various pain syndromes. Clinical management and subsequent rehabilitation are dependent upon accurate clinical assessment of the pain producing structures and a clinical impression to guide management.

The process begins early during undergraduate training that includes reasonably accurate anatomical landmark location of the extremity joints, related structures and associated soft tissues. It is also important to begin appreciating active and passive ranges of motion of the extremity joints plus the differences related to the quality of their clinical significance.

This chapter will introduce hard and soft landmark location of the shoulder, elbow and wrist/hand articulations of the upper extremity. The chapter will also demonstrate a number of rudimentary passive joint play procedures for the major joints of the upper extremity. This will introduce the student to appreciate normal extremity joint play and begin to develop the skills of joint analysis.

Section 1 Shoulder girdle

Section 1 will cover the shoulder girdle complex

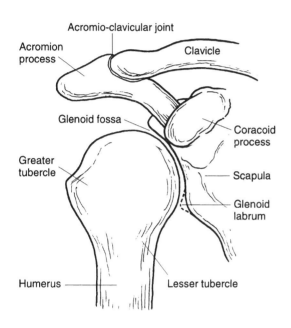

Acromion process
Acromio-clavicular joint
Clavicle
Glenoid fossa
Coracoid process
Greater tubercle
Scapula
Glenoid labrum
Humerus
Lesser tubercle

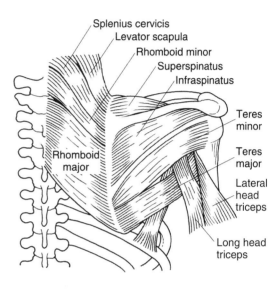

Splenius cervicis
Levator scapula
Rhomboid minor
Superspinatus
Infraspinatus
Rhomboid major
Teres minor
Teres major
Lateral head triceps
Long head triceps

SITTING POSITION

Many of the primary anatomical landmarks of the shoulder girdle are shown in Figure 7.1. These represent the major osseous landmarks targeted during visual and physical examination of this region.

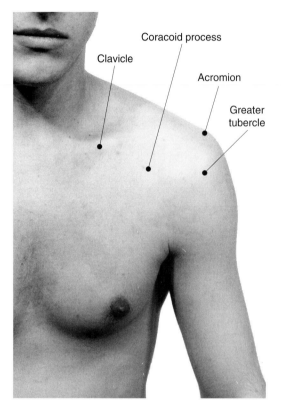

Coracoid process
Clavicle
Acromion
Greater tubercle

Fig. 7.1

Sternoclavicular joint (SC)

i)   With your finger feel the top edge of the manubrium as it concaves downward. This concavity (Figure 7.2) is known as the suprasternal (jugular) notch. Move laterally and feel the small tubercle of bone on the superior side at the proximal end of the clavicle. Now move down slightly and press posteriorly over the joint space to feel the elastic 'give' in the sternoclavicular capsular ligament.

Clavicle

i)   Continue to palpate along the length of the clavicle (Figure 7.3) to its distal attachment. The clavicle has both a concave and convex palpable section that should become evident during palpation.

ii) As you continue to palpate laterally along the clavicle it becomes more concave anteriorly just before the clavicle articulates with the acromion at the acromioclavicular joint (Figure 7.4).

Acromioclavicular joint (AC joint)

i)   Figure 7.5 demonstrates some of the anatomical landmarks located at the lateral shoulder region.

ii) With your finger(s) pressing from the superior part of the joint, note that the more prominent bump is the superior and lateral tubercle on the distal end of the clavicle

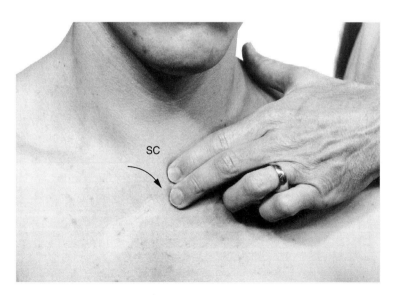

SC

Fig. 7.2

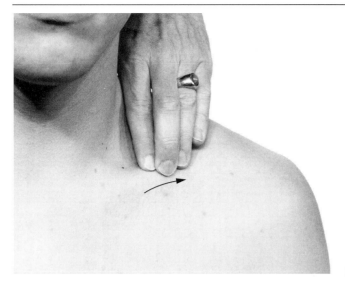

Fig. 7.3

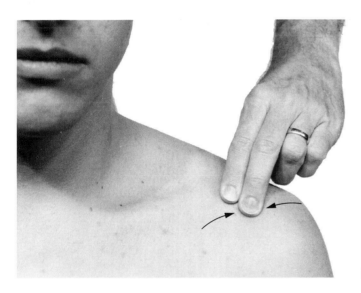

Fig. 7.4

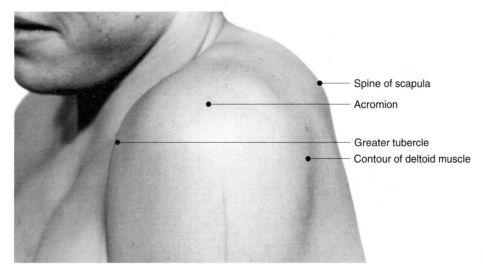

Spine of scapula

Acromion

Greater tubercle

Contour of deltoid muscle

Fig. 7.5

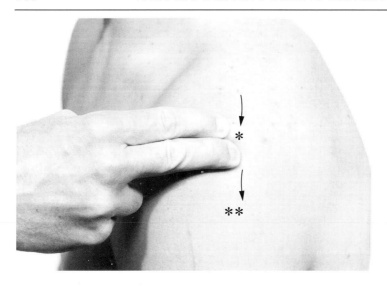

Fig. 7.6

(Figure 7.6). Move over this tubercle laterally and you will drop down onto the acromion. The acromion is best palpated with pressure both downward (inferior) and posteriorly. Use one finger tip to feel for the joint space (*), remembering to press gently. The superior A-C ligament is best felt with the palpating finger from the top (superiorly). You should be able to locate the lateral border of the acromion just lateral to the joint space. Continue to move laterally from the AC joint and palpate the deltoid muscle mass (**).

Acromion

i)   While standing beside your partner, the acromion can be felt along its superior surface as it curls back medially as an outward projection

of the scapula. Move back up superiorly and medially and identify the bony contour of the acromion as it becomes the scapular spine, while moving your fingers posteriorly (Figure 7.7).

ii) Now stand behind and move your fingers back to the acromion and continue laterally and down in front of the shoulder to locate the bulk of the deltoid muscle and the greater tubercle of the humerus (Figure 7.8).

Greater tubercle of the humerus

i)   With the arm slightly externally rotated and at rest feel for the larger bump on the outside edge of the upper portion of the humerus (Figure 7.9). This is a common insertion for the rotator cuff muscles of the shoulder and a

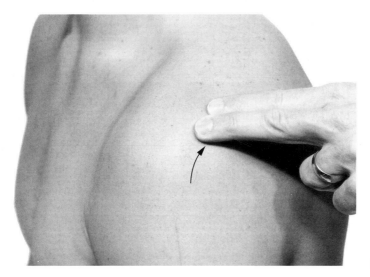

Fig. 7.7

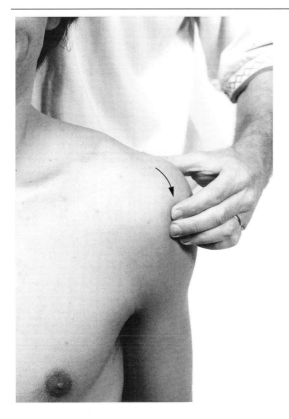

Fig. 7.8

typical region for clinical pain due to overuse sports injuries involving throwing. With your finger gently move medially and posteriorly down into the bicipital groove.

Bicipital groove (BG)

i) From the groove palpate medially and feel various soft tissue structures, including anterior deltoid fibres, tendon of the pectoralis anterior and the subacromial bursa (Figure 7.10). There is a small ligament which stabilizes the long head of the biceps muscle in the bicipital groove which is very difficult to palpate, but have a go! With your fingertip in the bicipital groove ask the patient to resist elbow flexion with your other hand offering resistance to the supinated forearm. You will feel the tendon of the biceps long head contract and develop tension. When flaccid, carefully feel again for the tubercle forming both sides of the bicipital groove.

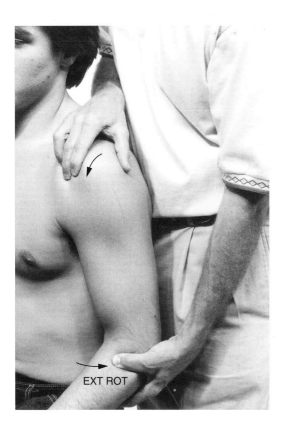

EXT ROT

Fig. 7.9

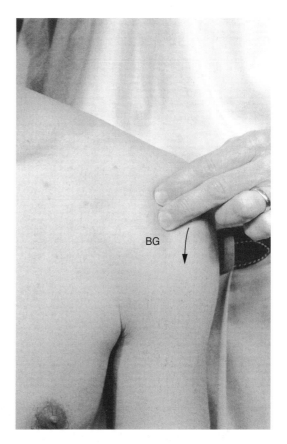

BG

Fig. 7.10

Lesser tubercle of the humerus

i) Feel more medially from the greater tubercle across the groove for the lesser tubercle, the inside border of the groove, which is more difficult to palpate but delineates the extent of the bicipital groove (Figure 7.11).

Coracoid process (CP)

i) Move back up to the acromion. Find the A-C joint space and drop the fingers down and slightly medially. Pressing through the anterior deltoid and pectoral fibres you will feel the coracoid as a spherical structure about the size of a golf ball under a layer of soft tissue (Figure 7.12).

ii) This area is the attachment point for a number of anterior shoulder girdle muscles including the pectoralis minor (*) and short head of the biceps (**). They can be palpated by running the palpating fingers laterally across the belly of the muscles (Figure 7.13).

MUSCULAR LANDMARKS

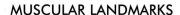

i) With your partner's cooperation, palpate these muscles both at rest and in various stages of gentle contraction.

Sternocleidomastoid (SCM)

i) The SCM is located on the anterolateral aspect of the cervical spine (Figure 7.14). Palpate the muscle in a relaxed state and under tension by creating slight resistance with one hand to the side of the jaw with your partner turning the head away from the SCM being examined. The SCM can be prominently palpated at both its clavicular (*) and mastoid (**) attachments.

Trapezius (upper portion)

i) Ask your partner to shrug the shoulder girdle, which contracts the large upper trapezius muscle (Figure 7.15). This can be palpated on top of the shoulder region as it nears its insertion on the scapular spine. This muscle should be palpated bilaterally as all soft tissue structures. This has clinical importance, particularly when assessing various pain syndromes related to the shoulder region.

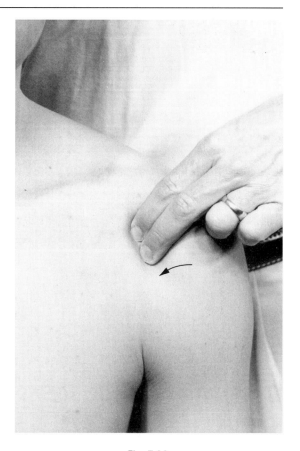

Fig. 7.11

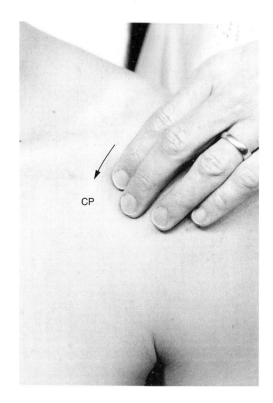

Fig. 7.12

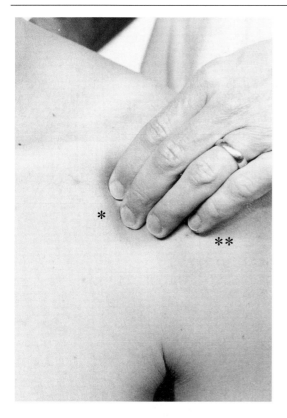

Fig. 7.13

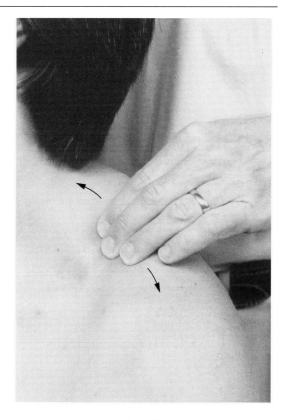

Fig. 7.15

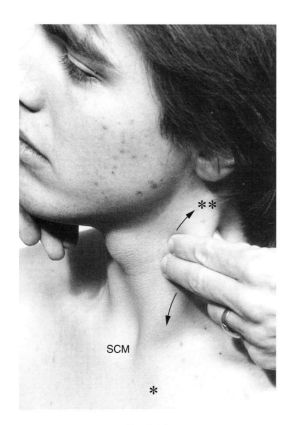

Fig. 7.14

Pectoralis major (PM)

i) Ask your partner to place the palms together and gently push to contract. Feel for both the origin of the PM at the costosternal junction (Figure 7.16) (*) and the narrower insertion into the bicipital groove (**). The bulk of the muscle mass makes up the anterior axillary fold.

Biceps brachii (long head) (BBL)

i) With the arm elevated and externally rotated simultaneously ask your partner to resist elbow flexion with the forearm slightly supinated. Use your palpating thumb to palpate the long head of the biceps at the musculotendinous junction (Figure 7.17). Palpate both heads of the biceps in their attachments on the anterior shoulder.

Biceps brachii (short head) (BBS)

i) Maintain the arm in the same posture as Figure 7.17 and palpate more posteriorly to appreciate the short head of biceps using the palpating

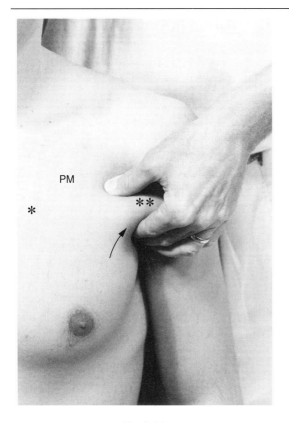

Fig. 7.16

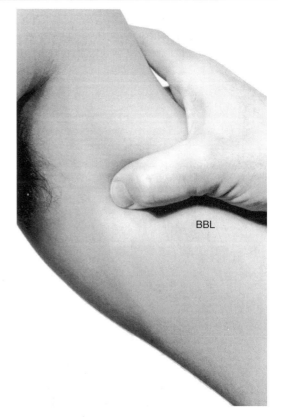

Fig. 7.18

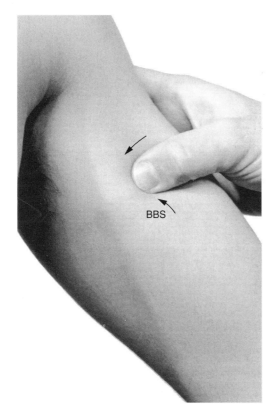

Fig. 7.17

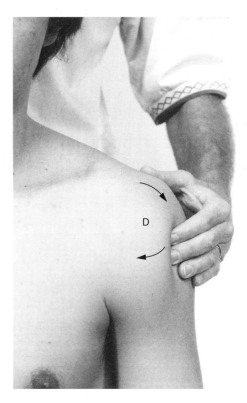

Fig. 7.19

thumb (Figure 7.18). These are difficult to palpate but slightly easier when under resistance. Keep in mind the clinical perspective with these structures.

Deltoid (D)

i)   From the acromion move laterally and slightly inferior to feel the anterior, middle and posterior deltoid fibres (Figure 7.19). Because this muscle wraps around the shoulder, its three parts can be contracted separately by offering slight resistance to the arm in flexion, extension or abduction. Position yourself at various positions around your partner to feel this muscle's parts contract. Distinguish deltoid fibres from the others in the bicipital groove and the anterior axillary fold noted above.

FUNDAMENTAL JOINT PLAY SKILLS OF THE SHOULDER GIRDLE COMPLEX

Developing the ability to appreciate the subtle natural spring and compliance associated with the individual synovial joints of the shoulder girdle is a necessary pre-manipulative skill. Though the upper limb has a wide range of global motion in various complex axes and planes, it is the passive joint play of the individual articulations that collectively contributes to this overall function. The shoulder girdle is a very complex system of multiple joints offering a wide range of flexibility in all ranges. There is however a question regarding overall stability which is compromised due to the inherent flexibility.

Learning to appreciate subtle passive involuntary motion of the major articulations of the shoulder girdle complex is a prerequisite for assessment and mobilization and/or manipulative intervention. These skills are similar to those presented in the previous chapters and constitute basic psychomotor acquisition and joint analysis procedures. At this point in undergraduate training applying new anatomical landmark location and palpation skills requires clinical application and frameworking.

This section presents an overview of rudimentary joint play skills for the shoulder girdle complex. Emphasis is placed upon reasonable anatomical accuracy, joint location, posture and joint play challenge motor skills. Importance will be placed upon introducing an appropriate amount of force across or along the respective joints to engage the natural spring or compliance that is an inherent feature of all synovial joints. Factors such as joint architecture,

surrounding holding elements and axes of motion will all influence joint play magnitudes and performance. Keep in mind that normal joint play or spring in a neutral position is extremely small and subtle. It is an appreciation of the natural give or flexibility of all synovial/diarthroidial joints and is necessary for optimal joint function. The amount of joint play varies depending on the specific joint characteristics. This is a reasonable reference point to begin assimilating these motor skills and appreciation.

Supine position joint play

i)   Place your partner supine on the table and stand on the ipsilateral side of the table facing your patient. Hold the arm in slight flexion and place the thenar eminence of the left hand over the anterolateral aspect of the humeral head (Figure 7.20). Note the sternal notch position to target joint (*).

ii) Apply a gentle compression posteriorly (downward) to introduce a neutral joint play movement of the glenohumeral joint (Figure 7.21). Feel the motion of the head of the humerus back and forth in the glenohumeral joint, this being anterior to posterior glide.

iii) With the same hand positions, gently pull back (inferiorly) with the examiner's inferior hand (holding the wrist) to feel a gentle stretching

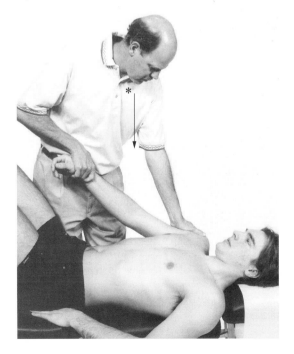

Fig. 7.20

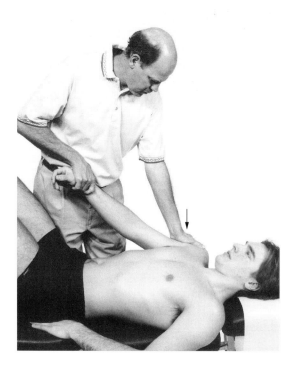

Fig. 7.21

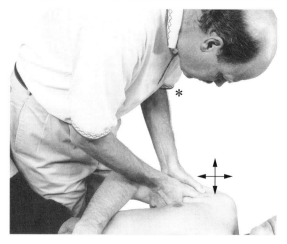

Fig. 7.23

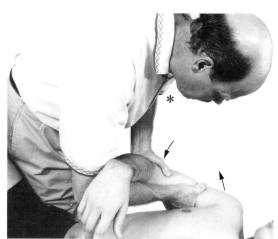

Fig. 7.24

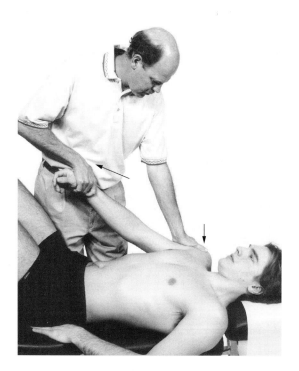

Fig. 7.22

motion at the glenohumeral joint, this motion is termed long axis distraction (Figure 7.22).

iv) Bend down and grasp the upper end of the humerus with both hands (Figure 7.23). When the hands are opposed and the arm firmly held, move them together in a posterior to anterior and then a superior and inferior direction. These movements are termed anterior-posterior and superior-inferior joint play. This multiaxial joint play procedure can also be performed in the prone position. Note the sternal notch position (*).

v) Next move the outside hand down towards the elbow and push the upper hand in the axilla laterally outward to feel slight lateral movement at the glenohumeral joint. This is lateral gapping (Figure 7.24). This joint play procedure can also be performed in the prone posture. Note the position of the sternal notch (*).

SUMMARY

This section has presented an overview of the palpation methods required to locate major anatomical landmarks of the shoulder girdle. A basic introduction to a variety of fundamental joint play procedures and joint assessment skills has also been presented. It is up to the student to pursue acquiring and developing these skills as a prerequisite to advancing their training to include various manipulative psychomotor skills that are introduced later in the educational curriculum.

Section 2 The elbow

This section will cover the elbow

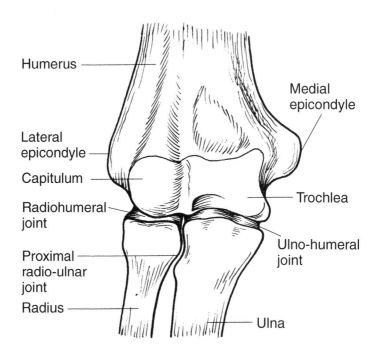

Humerus

Medial epicondyle

Lateral epicondyle

Capitulum

Trochlea

Radiohumeral joint

Ulno-humeral joint

Proximal radio-ulnar joint

Radius

Ulna

Medial Epicondyle

i) Figures 7.25 and 7.26 illustrate some of the important anatomical landmarks located on the medial and posterior aspects of the elbow, respectively.

ii) Stand beside your partner from behind and hold the front of the arm with your hand (same side) slightly abducting and flexing the joint. With your other hand, use your thumb and index finger to palpate the large bumpy protrusion on the inside of the arm.

This is the medial epicondyle (ME), part of the lower end of the humerus (Figure 7.27). This is the most visible and palpable osseous landmark on the medial aspect of the elbow. The ME can be found by either palpating from above or below the elbow. The ME functions as the common flexor tendon attachment, which has a number of clinical implications. Learn to palpate bilaterally in order to make subtle comparisons both sides.

iii) Now move around to face your partner and switch your hands to palpate that same side medial epicondyle with the thumb and first finger of your other hand (Figure 7.28). Palpate and appreciate the identifiable landmarks above and below the epicondyles using both thumb and fingers. Continue to palpate slightly superiorly, feeling for the contour of the epicondyle as it smooths out into the shaft of the humerus, and then further up as it is covered by triceps muscle travelling superiorly (*). From the epicondyle, move distally and feel the muscular bulk of the wrist flexors.

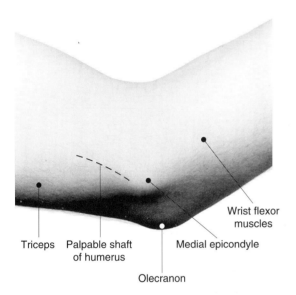

Fig. 7.25

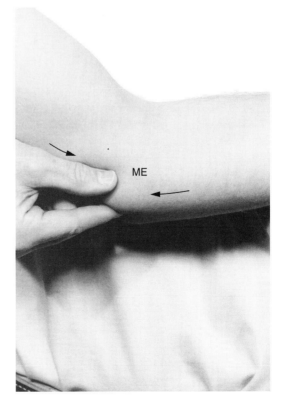

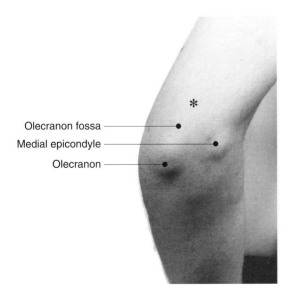

Fig. 7.26   Fig. 7.27

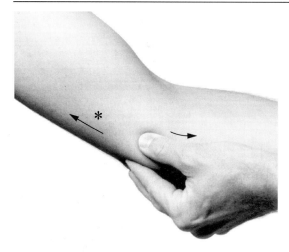

Fig. 7.28

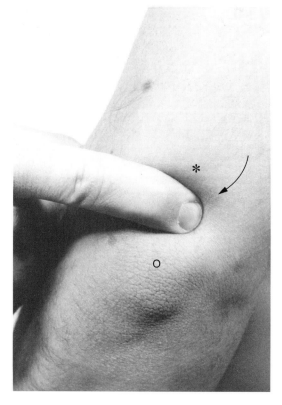

Fig. 7.29

Olecranon (O)

i) Posteriorly, the largest protuberance is the ole-
    cranon, *the proximal end of the ulna* (Figure 7.26).
    With the joint in anatomical position and with
    the musculature at complete rest, feel for the
    fossa, the indentation just above the tip of the
    olecranon, and note the elastic feel of the tri-
    ceps tendon (Figure 7.29) (*). Apply light
    pressure with the tip of the palpating finger
    over the olecranon fossa to appreciate more
    fully the soft tissues in the region and more
    specifically the common triceps tendon (*). If
    your partner contracts the muscle slightly
    against resistance into extension you will feel
    the muscle fibres contract and the tension
    develop in the tendon.

ii) Move the elbow joint into full flexion and
    with the other hand feel the movement of
    the olecranon through this range of motion
    from extension to flexion (Figure 7.30).
    Appreciate the tissue laxity in full extension
    and the ability to palpate the olecranon and
    related soft tissues compared to the changes
    at full flexion. This region also has clinical
    significance, particularly the olecranon
    bursa, which lies over the olecranon itself
    (*).

iii) With the elbow in full flexion place the thumb
    pad over the lateral epicondyle (Figure 7.31)
    (*) and the index finger over the medial epi-
    condyle (**). In full flexion these two struc-
    tures, plus the olecranon, form a triangular
    shape which has important clinical implica-
    tions.

Lateral epicondyle (LE)

i) From the olecranon move laterally to the tip of
    the lateral epicondyle (LE) with the thumb
    pad. Support the elbow with the palpating
    hand. The LE is the attachment for the com-
    mon extensor tendon, which has a number of
    important clinical implications, particularly
    tennis elbow (Figure 7.32). Locate and

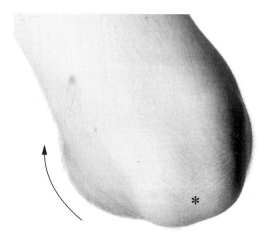

Fig. 7.30

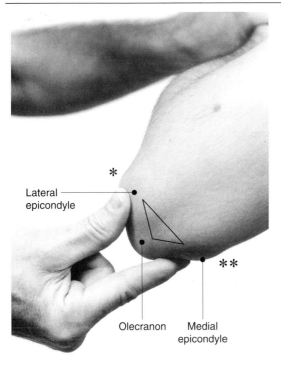

Fig. 7.31

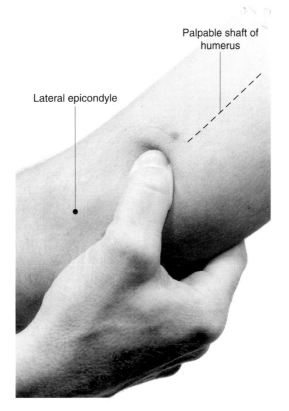

Fig. 7.33

appreciate the extensor muscles as they attach to the LE (*).

ii) Moving upward (proximally) you will feel the lateral supracondylar ridge of the humerus which is felt for about one third of the length of the humerus with increasing muscular thickness before the bone is no longer directly palpable due to the increase in overlying muscle (Figure 7.33).

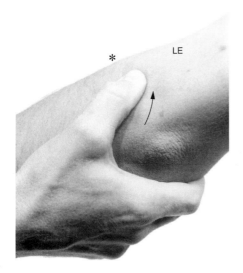

Fig. 7.32

iii) From the lateral epicondyle move slightly distally and your finger will drop into a very slight depression which is the radiohumeral joint. The capitullum is the articulating process of the humerus. The overlying tissue has an elastic feel, this being the radiohumeral ligament (Figure 7.34). By pronating and supinating the wrist, the palpator should be able to appreciate movement of this joint as well as feel the fibrous ligamentous tissue.

iv) Immediately below this is the radial head, which should be felt as a smaller bump compared to the epicondyle. Active and passive forearm supination and pronation will rotate the radial head (Figure 7.35). The palpator should be able to appreciate the movement of the radial head and the fibrous annular ligament. Use both your thumb and index finger to feel the movement of the radial head (*).

v) Move your fingers down distally from the lateral epicondyle to palpate the belly of the extensors of the wrist and hand (Figure 7.36). Ask your partner to offer slight resistance to your support hand in extension at the

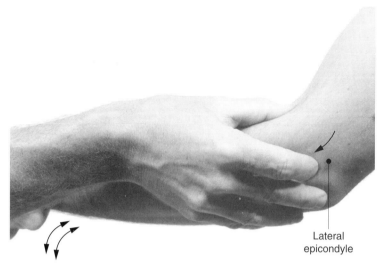

Lateral
epicondyle

Fig. 7.34

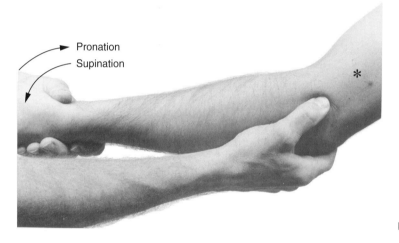

Pronation

Supination

*

Fig. 7.35

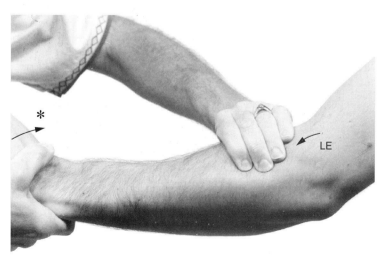

*

LE

Fig. 7.36

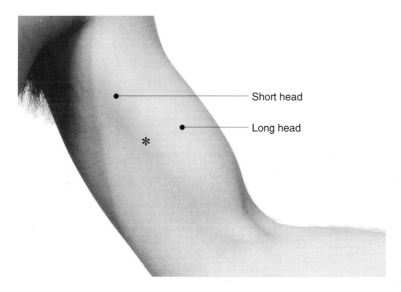

Short head

Long head

*

Fig. 7.37

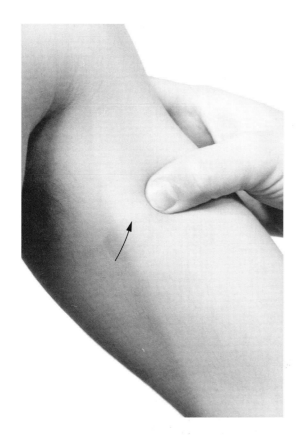

Fig. 7.38

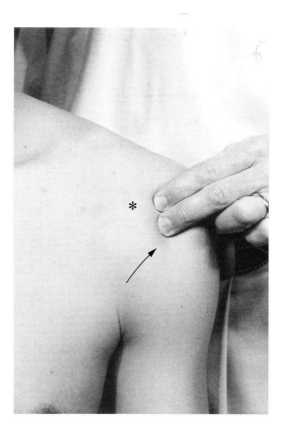

*

Fig. 7.39

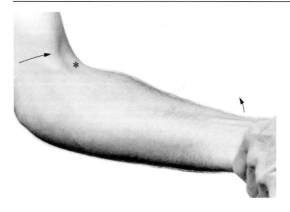

Fig. 7.40

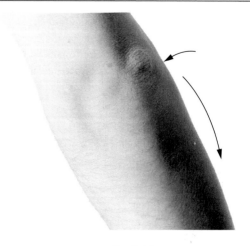

Fig. 7.42

wrist to feel these muscles contract (*). This will permit the examiner to appreciate the bulk of the muscles and their attachment point at the LE.

Biceps brachii (BB)

i)   The short head of the biceps originates from the coracoid process and is palpable with slight contraction and relaxation from your partner (Figure 7.37). The belly of the short head is best felt at the mid-humerus point on the inside of the arm (*).

ii) Palpate posteriorly and laterally to the more prominent belly of the long head, as the muscle is contracted by resisting flexion at the elbow (Figure 7.38). The biceps muscle has important clinical implications particularly with respect to sports-related injuries.

iii) The long head of biceps can be palpated up to its origin and passes through the bicipital groove superiorly up to the supraglenoid tubercle (of the scapula) (Figure 7.39). The

specific attachment is difficult to palpate as the deltoid fibres cover it (*).

iv) Distally, the long head is more prominent at the attachment point at the biceps tubercle on the ulna (*), especially when contracted against resistance by the patient (Figure 7.40).

v)   The long head of biceps tendon at its distal attachment can be easily palpated and assessed during forearm contraction (Figure 7.41). When your partner resists you as you gently pull down on the forearm and wrist, palpate both heads of the biceps and the wrist and finger flexors.

Ulna (U)

i)   From the olecranon (Figure 7.42) move distally and you can feel the sharp ridge of the ulna all the way down to its lower attachment at the distal radio-ulnar joint (Figure 7.43) which can be located with the palpating fingers (*).

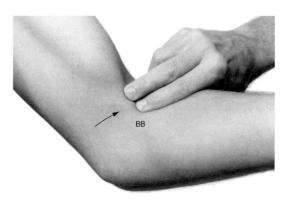

Fig. 7.41

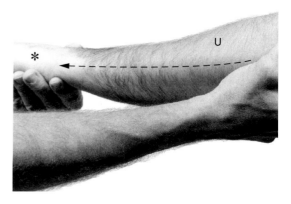

Fig. 7.43

SUMMARY

This section has presented an overview of the palpation methods required to locate major anatomical landmarks of the elbow including the forearm and upper arm regions. It is up to the student to pursue acquiring and developing these skills as a prerequisite to advancing their training to include various manipulative psychomotor skills that are introduced later in the educational curriculum.

Section 3 The wrist and hand

The section will cover the wrist and hand

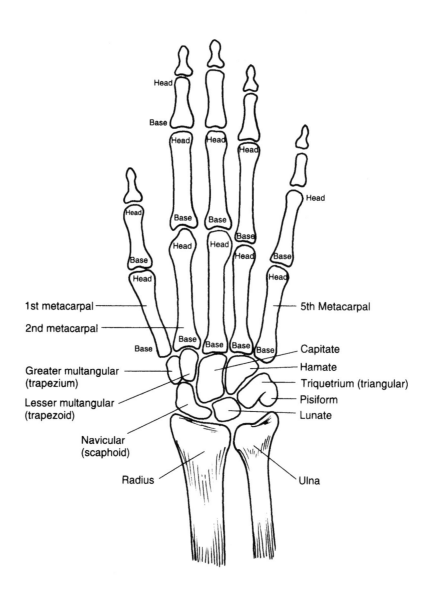

WRIST REGION

Dorsal structures

i) Figures 7.44 (*) left hand and 7.45 (**) right hand illustrate a number of important osseous landmarks and other anatomical structures located on the dorsum of the wrist. Note the proximity of the carpal bones in both the proximal and distal rows.

ii) Sit or stand facing your practice partner and lightly grasp the hand and wrist with both your hands wrapping the index fingers around to the volar surface to stabilize the grip (Figure 7.46) (*). This permits the use of both thumbs to palpate the dorsal landmarks (**).

iii) In order to palpate and identify the individual osseous structures of the proximal carpal row start by locating the radial styloid with the palpating thumbs (Figure 7.47) (*). From this position, which is best palpated on the lateral aspect, move the palpating thumbs distally to feel the joint depression between the styloid process and the scaphoid (navicular). Use the thumbs to map out the scaphoid. The scaphoid has clinical importance with respect to a common fracture site and poor healing properties.

iv) Move the palpating thumbs laterally towards the 5th digit along the same anatomical line to appreciate the joint lines and the next carpal structure, the lunate (Figure 7.48).

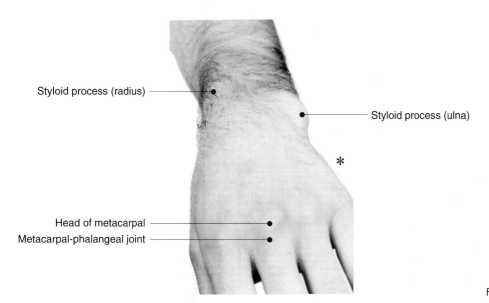

Styloid process (radius)

Styloid process (ulna)

*

Head of metacarpal
Metacarpal-phalangeal joint

Fig. 7.44

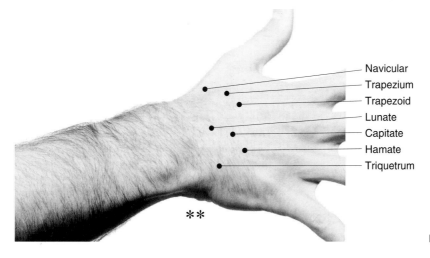

Navicular
Trapezium
Trapezoid
Lunate
Capitate
Hamate
Triquetrum

**

Fig. 7.45

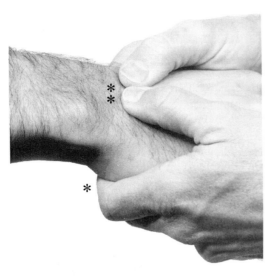

Fig. 7.46

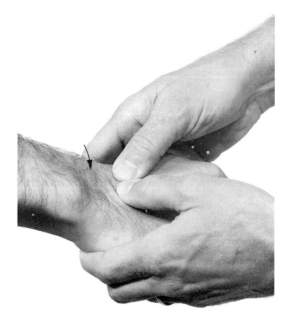

Fig. 7.48

v) Continue to move laterally towards the 5th digit across the dorsum of the hand and appreciate various joint lines until the most lateral component of the proximal row is encountered, the triquetrum (Figure 7.49a). The pisiform is located just under the triquetrum, which can be palpated and located by the index finger (*). *Learn to visualize these structures during palpation.* The carpal joints are cov-

ered by ligaments which are very thin and, when gently pressed with the thumb or finger, give with a slight elastic feel. The tendons are also elastic in nature but are thicker and have a round contour. The triquetrum may be palpated using thumb pads positioned side by side as with the other proximal row structures (Figure 7.49b).

vi) Move the palpating thumbs distally to the distal row of carpal bones beginning just distal to the scaphoid (navicular). The first osseous structure is the trapezium followed by the trapezoid, capitate *(located directly distal to the tubercle positioned at the distal aspect of the radius)* and the hamate (Figure 7.50) (*).

vii) With the palpating fingers located at the radiocarpal junction move the wrist/hand into flexion (palm down) to appreciate the movement of the proximal row of carpal bones as they articulate at the distal end of the radius (Figure 7.51).

viii) With the palpating fingers in the same position, move the thumbs just distal to appreciate the mid-carpal joint (locate the capitate) and extend (dorsum up) the wrist/hand to appreciate extension of the mid-carpal joints (Figure 7.52). These joint structures have clinical significance, particularly following sports-related injuries. Identify each carpal by using both thumbs and moving the wrist back and forth in flexion-extension and radial-ulnar

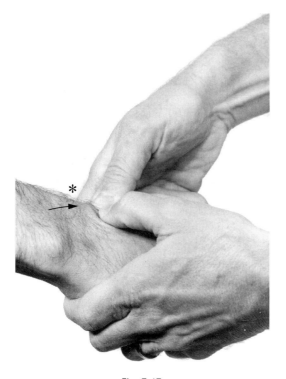

Fig. 7.47

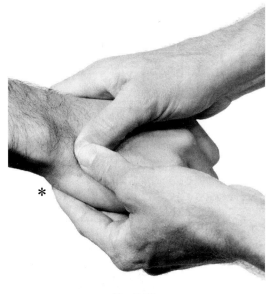

Fig. 7.49a

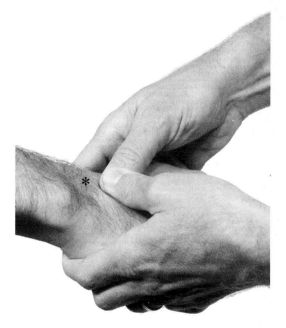

Fig. 7.50

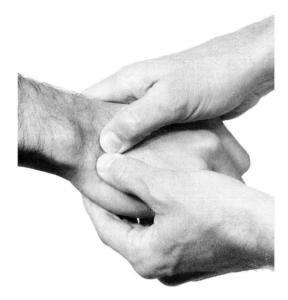

Fig. 7.49b

wrist laterally in radial and ulnar deviation in order to appreciate the movement of the carpal structures during lateral joint play. Appreciate the elastic give associated with this movement. This may be lost in mechanical pain conditions that present clinically.

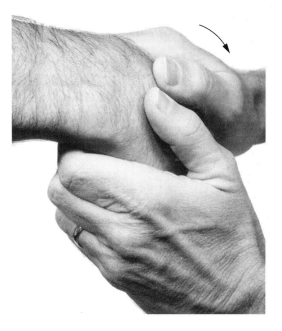

deviation. Feel the difference between the capsular ligaments of the carpal-to-carpal joints, which are very thin, and the carpal-wrist joints, which are thicker.

ix) On the ulnar side, the prominent bump dorsally is the ulnar styloid (Figure 7.53) (*). Move distally and feel the elastic quality to the soft tissues here: the more superficial tendon is the *extensor carpi ulnaris* and deep to this, feel the ulnar collateral ligament which joins the ulna to the triquetrum. Now move the

Fig. 7.51

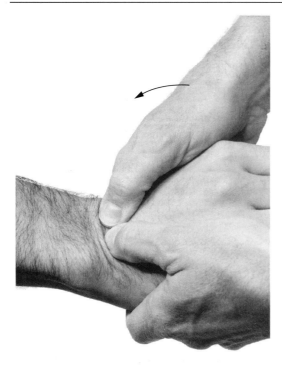

Fig. 7.52

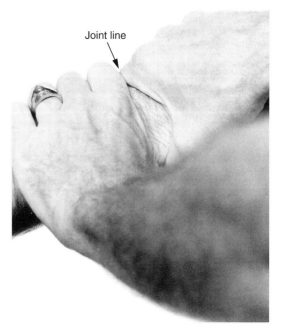

Joint line

Fig. 7.54

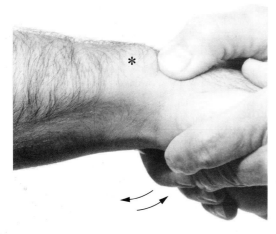

Fig. 7.53

JOINT PLAY MOTION PROCEDURES

A-P shear radiocarpal joint

i) Stand beside your partner and grasp the hand
and forearm at the wrist (Figure 7.54) just
firmly enough to move the wrist joint in a
shearing motion up and down. Keep the
hands and arms straight and move them in
opposite directions moving back and forth
from the shoulders. This is anterior-posterior

shear (Figure 7.55). Appreciate the passive
involuntary elasticity associated with normal
joint motion. This A-P shear can be reproduced for the mid-carpal joint. Keep in mind
the small amount of inherent give in the joint.
Some individuals will be slightly more flexible
than others so always compare joint play bilaterally. Note the sternal notch (*), relative to
the joint being assessed.

Long axis distraction – joint play

Radiocarpal joint

i) With your same hand position as in Figure
7.55, bend your arms comfortably and gently
pull the hands apart separating the wrist joint.
Repeat this motion several times in order to
appreciate the natural tissue elasticity (Figure
7.56). This is long axis distraction (also called
long axis extension) of the radiocarpal joint
(wrist). Compare joint play on both sides, as
they should, under normal conditions, be very
similar. This will be quite the opposite during
clinical presentations.

Wrist joint – palmar

i) Figure 7.57 illustrates the major osseous landmarks identifiable from the palmar surface of
the wrist region.

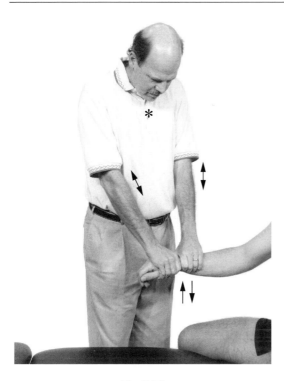

Fig. 7.55

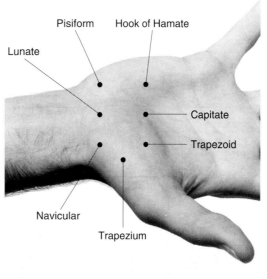

Fig. 7.57

ii) Using the same finger and thumb pad configuration as the dorsum of the hand begin to identify the structures illustrated in Figure 7.57. Begin at the radial side and move laterally towards the ulnar side (5th digit) from the navicular (scaphoid) to the triquetrum and then back along the distal row to the radial side and the trapezium (Figure 7.58).

iii) On the radial aspect feel the prominent styloid process at the end of the radius. Move over the bump distally and feel the elastic give on the radial collateral ligament (Figure 7.59).

iv) Move slightly laterally (radially) and feel the tendon of the *abductor pollicis longus* (Figure 7.60) (*), which is easily felt when resistance to abduction against the thumb is produced.

v) If your partner moves the thumb into abduction and deviates the wrist radially, the *anatomical snuff box* is created by the *abductor pollicis longus* tendon on the anterior side and the tendon of the *extensor pollicis longus* on the dorsal or posterior side (Figure 7.61). These structures have clinical importance particularly after trauma.

vi) Push down into the groove or floor of the snuff box and palpate the navicular (scaphoid) (Figure 7.62). The scaphoid is a commonly fractured bone in the hand and requires early detection and appropriate management in order to ensure restoration of overall function of this part of the hand. The palpator can apply a little joint play force through this region to appreciate the joint give.

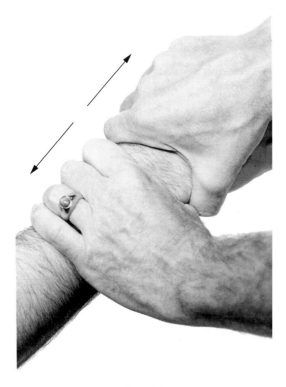

Fig. 7.56

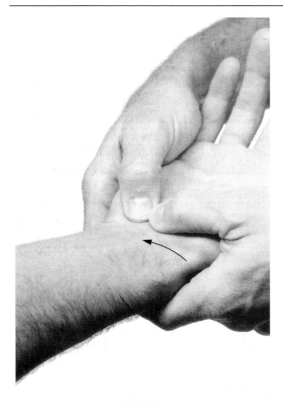

Fig. 7.58

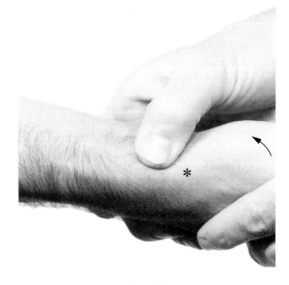

Fig. 7.60

vii) Move back to the palmar surface and feel the anterior wrist joint (Figure 7.63). The flexor tendons are palpable both at rest and with slight flexion contraction.

viii) The navicular is felt on the distal side of the wrist joint when you move from the first metacarpal to the midline of the wrist. It is a palpable bump at the proximal end of the thenar eminence (Figure 7.64) (*).

ix) On the other side of the anterior/palmar wrist, the pisiform is the bump at the proximal end of the hypothenar eminence (Figure 7.65)

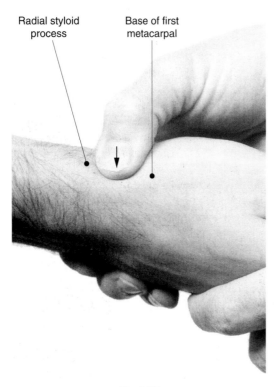

Radial styloid process

Base of first metacarpal

Fig. 7.59

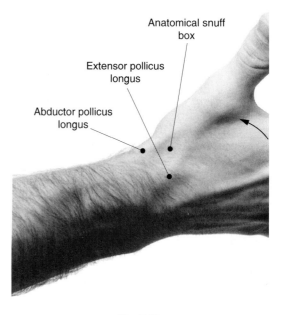

Anatomical snuff box

Extensor pollicus longus

Abductor pollicus longus

Fig. 7.61

(*), this being the small muscle mass on the ulnar side of the palm. These structures plus the thenar eminence have important roles in chiropractic manipulative skills as contact points on anatomical levers.

Metacarpals

i)   The five metacarpals are more easily palpated on the dorsum of the hand because the palmar hand muscles cover the anterior bones. With your partner's hand at rest, squeeze gently to compress the hand, feeling the contours of the metacarpals and the soft tissues between them (Figure 7.66).

ii) Now press your thumbs more firmly to feel along the length of the shaft of each metacarpal. Move distally to the five prominent distal enlargements of the metacarpals (Figure 7.67a).

iii) The metacarpophalangeal joints (*) are spaces felt by pressing through the more superficial tissues: the tendons inserting on each digit, both on the palmar and dorsal surfaces (Figure 7.67b). These joints are small and

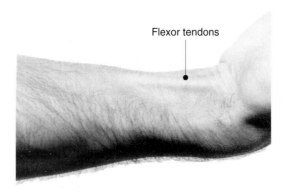

Fig. 7.63

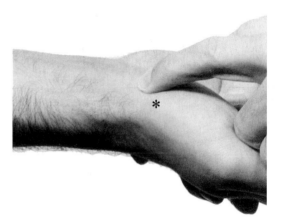

Fig. 7.64

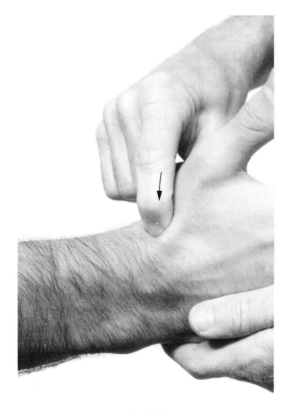

Fig. 7.62

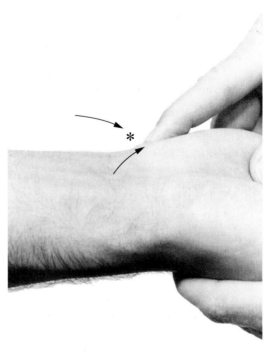

Fig. 7.65

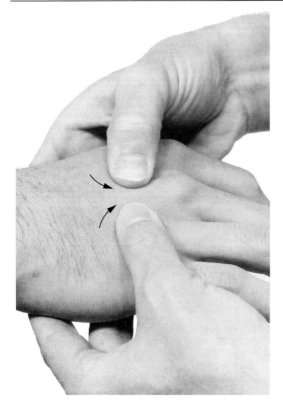

Fig. 7.66

flat and therefore difficult to appreciate but have clinical significance.

Palmar surface of the hand

i)   By having your partner contract the thumb and finger flexors against opposite resistance, you will be able to visualize the thenar and hypothenar muscle eminences, and feel the flexor tendons to the thumb and fingers (Figure 7.68).

ii) By resisting abduction or ulnar deviation of the 5th metatarsal the lateral border of the hypothenar eminence becomes more prominent (Figure 7.69) (*).

Thumb

i)   Figure 7.70 illustrates flexion of the first metacarpophalangeal (*) and first interphalangeal joint (**) of the thumb. Also note and palpate the corresponding tendons related to thumb function, which is multidimensional and important clinically.

ii) Palpate the length of the thumb from the first metacarpal at the wrist along past the first metacarpophalangeal joint (Figure 7.71) (*) across the proximal phalange to the interphalangeal joint (**) and to the distal phalange.

iii) Figure 7.72 illustrates palpation and location of the interphalangeal joint of the thumb (*).

Joint play of the thumb

i)   Grasp the first metacarpal at the proximal end with thumb and forefinger (Figure 7.73) (*) and the other hand firmly around carpal structures, particularly the trapezium (**).

ii) The palpator stands at the side of the patient with the wrist firmly gripped and the sternal notch positioned over the structures being assessed (Figure 7.74).

iii) Gently pull or distract the first carpometacarpal joint straight out being careful not to twist or bend (Figure 7.75). Feel the give through the joint. This joint play motion can also be done with the examiner sitting or standing. Try to maintain good posture and body alignment during this procedure.

iv) This particular procedure may be used to assess a number of joints along this kinetic chain including the metacarpophalangeal and interphalangeal joints by moving the contacts accordingly (Figure 7.76). *The important skill is to get the opposing hand contacts as close to the targeted joint as possible to isolate a specific joint complex, to avoid any extraneous tissue or joint movement which may confound the procedure.*

Joint play of the fingers

i)   Move distally along each finger's three phalanges and feel the interphalangeal joints (Figure 7.77) (*). Palpate the shaft and small end bump (tubercle) of each phalange for all four fingers.

Finger joint play

i)   Using the thumb and forefinger grasp the proximal phalanx at the metacarpal-phalangeal joint for each finger (Figure 7.78) (*). Then grasp the distal metacarpal of each finger with the thumb and other fingers on the palmar aspect (**). This will isolate the targeted joint and ensure that joint play forces are directed at a single joint.

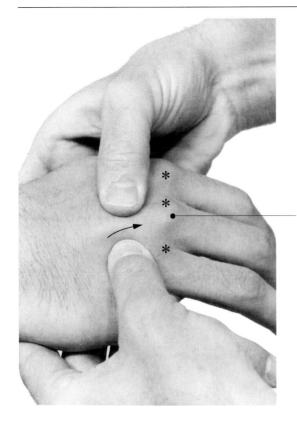

Third metacarpal-
phalangeal joint

Fig. 7.67a

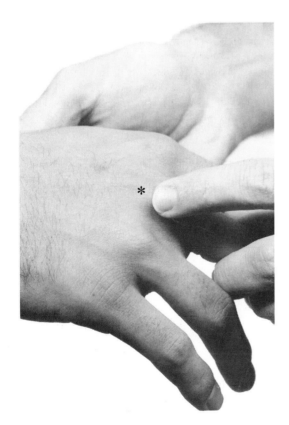

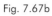

Fig. 7.67b

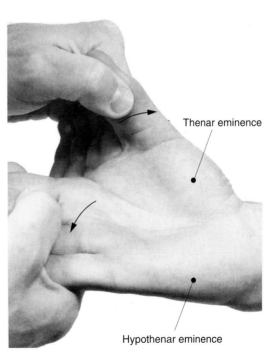

Thenar eminence

Hypothenar eminence

Fig. 7.68

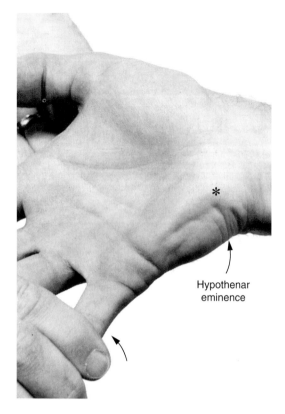

Hypothenar
eminence

Fig. 7.69

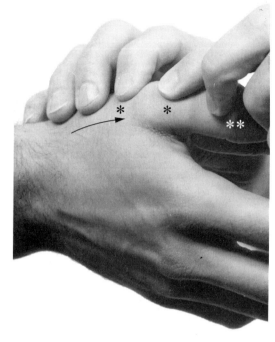

Fig. 7.71

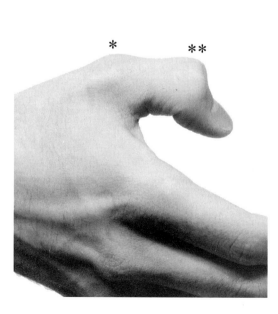

Fig. 7.70

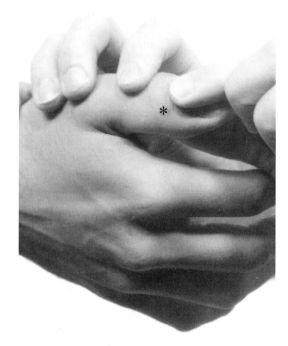

Fig. 7.72

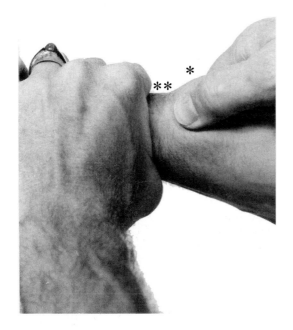

Fig. 7.73

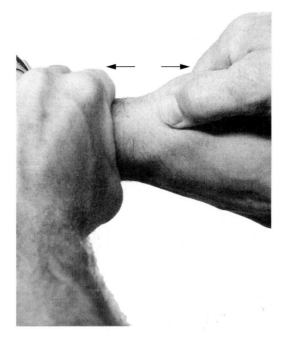

Fig. 7.75

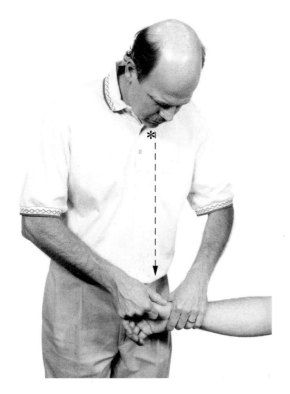

Fig. 7.74

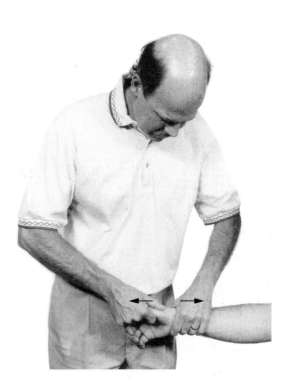

Fig. 7.76

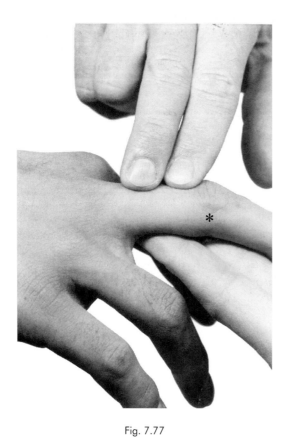

Fig. 7.77

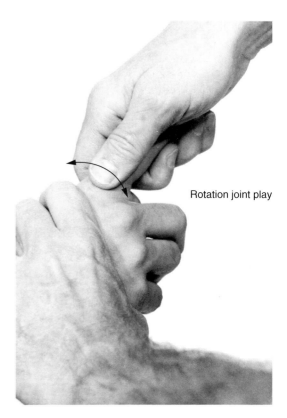

Fig. 7.79

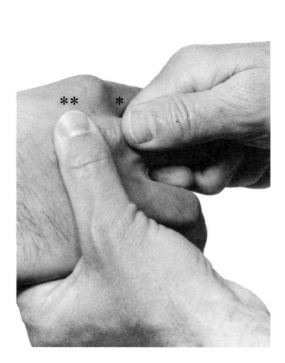

Fig. 7.78

Fig. 7.80

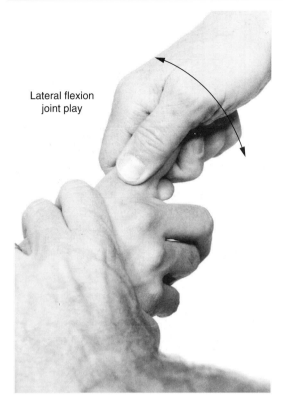

Lateral flexion
joint play

Fig. 7.81

ii) Distract the distal contact in order to assess the long axis joint play of the 3rd metacarpophalangeal joint (Figure 7.79). Maintain stability (S) of one hand to appreciate joint separation.

iii) This procedure can be repeated to test other planes of motion including rotation (Figure 7.80) and lateral flexion (gapping) (Figure 7.81). Each finger's metacarpal and interphalangeal joints can be moved in the passive range of motion. This should be repeated for all joints and bilaterally.

SUMMARY

This section has presented an overview of the palpation methods required to locate major anatomical landmarks of the wrist and hand. This has also included a basic introduction to a variety of fundamental joint play procedures and joint assessment skills. It is up to the student to pursue acquiring and developing these skills as a prerequisite to advancing their training to include various manipulative psychomotor skills that are introduced later in the educational curriculum.

FURTHER READING

Bergmann, T., Peterson, D., Lawrence, D. (1993) *Chiropractic Technique*. Churchill Livingstone, London.

Byfield, D. (1996) *Chiropractic Manipulative Skills*. Butterworth-Heinemann, Oxford.

Magee, D. (1987) *Orthopaedic Physical Assessment*. W.B. Saunders Company, London.

Index

Abductor pollicis longus, 159, 160
Acetabulum, 126
Achilles tendon, 94, 95, 103, 105
Achilles tendon insertion, 94, 95
Acromioclavicular joint, 135, 136–8
Acromion process, 135, 136, 138
Active motion palpation, 4–8
Adductor tubercle, 114, 115
Anatomical snuff box, 169
Anterior chest wall palpation, 74–5
Anterior cruciate ligament, 111
Anterior superior iliac spine, 127, 129
Anterior talofibular ligament, 103

Biceps brachii, 141–3, 151, 152
Biceps femoris, 118, 119
Bicipital groove, 139

Calcaneofibular ligament, 103
Calcaneus, 89
    lateral aspect, 97, 98
    medial aspect, 94, 95
Capitate, 154
Capitulum, 146
Cervicothoracic and occiput palpation, 79–85
    prone position, 81–5
    sitting palpation, 80–1
Clavicle, 135, 136
Coracoid process, 135, 136, 140
Counter-rotation specific joint play analysis, 61–3
Cuboid bone, 89, 96, 97
Cuneiform bone, 89, 92, 93

Degrees of freedom, 13–14
Deltoid ligament, 103
Deltoid muscle, 142, 143
Diagnostic palpation, 1–33
    clinical considerations and kinematics, 14
    clinical palpation methods, 2–12
        active/dynamic motion palpation, 4–8
        motion palpation, 3–4
        passive accessory palpation, 8–11
        static palpation, 2–6
    educational value, 22–5
    intervertebral joint fixation, 15

kinematics and motion palpation, 12–14
    degrees of freedom, 13–14
    kinematics versus kinetics, 12
    right-handed cartesian coordinate system, 12–13
    types of motion, 12, 13
motion palpation reliability/validity studies, 15–19
    reliability studies, 16–18
    validity studies, 18–19
segmental identification and specificity assumption,
    19–22
Dorsalis pedis artery, 105–6
Dynamic end play analysis
    pelvic complex and sacroiliac joint, 64–7
        lateral bending, 63–4
        reciprocal innominate movement, 64–5
        specific sacroiliac joint movement, 65–7
    thoracolumbar spine, 67–71
        combined movement end play, 71–2
        extension end play, 71
        lateral bending and play, 68–71
        recommended position for, 68–9
        rotation end play, 71
Dynamic motion palpation, 4–8
Dynamic postural examination
    sitting, 41–3
        forward flexion, 41–2
        lateral flexion, 41–3
    standing, 39–41
        backward extension, lateral view, 41
        forward flexion, lateral view, 39–41
        lateral flexion, posterior-anterior view, 41

Educational aspects, 22–5
Elastic zone, 10, 13
Elbow, 146–53
    biceps brachii, 151, 152
    lateral epicondyle, 148–52
    medial epicondyle, 147–8
    olecranon, 148
    ulna, 152
End feel, 11
End play, 11
    see also Dynamic end play analysis
Ethical issues, xvi–xvii
Extensor digitorum longus, 102

Extensor hallucis longus, 102
Extensor pollicis longus, 159, 161

Femoral condyle
    lateral, 116, 117
    medial, 113, 115
Femur, 126
Fibular head, 116, 117
Fingers, 162, 165–7
Foot and ankle palpation, 89–110
    active range of motion, 90–1
    joint play, 106–10
        intermetatarsal joint, 110
        metatarsophalangeal joint, 109–10
        subtalar joint, 109
        talocrural joint, 107–9
    lateral aspect, 96–9
        cuboid, 96–7
        fifth metatarsal and styloid process, 96
        fifth metatarsophalangeal joint, 96
        lateral calcaneus, 97
        lateral malleolus, 98–9
        superficial soft anatomical structures, 96
    medial aspect, 91–5
        Achilles tendon, 94, 95
        Achilles tendon insertion, 94, 95
        first (medial) cuneiform, 92, 93
        first metatarsophalangeal joint, 91
        head of talus, 92–3
        medial calcaneus, 94, 95
        medial malleolus, 94
        metatarsals, 91–2
        navicular, 92
        sustentaculum tali, 94, 95
    plantar aspect, 99–105
        Achilles tendon, 103, 105
        anterior talofibular ligament, 103
        calcaneofibular ligament, 103
        extensor digitorum longus, 102
        extensor hallucis longus, 102
        lateral collateral ligaments, 102–3
        medial collateral ligament, 103
        peroneus longus, 102
        soft tissue landmarks, 102–5
        tibialis anterior, 102
    vascular structures, 105–6
        dorsalis pedis artery, 105–6
        popliteal artery, 106
        posterior tibial artery, 106
Fovea capitis femoris, 126

Gastrocnemius, medial and lateral head, 119–20
Glenoid fossa, 135
Glenoid labrum, 135
Gluteus medius, 127, 129
Gracilis muscle, 120
Greater trochanter, 126, 127

Hamate bone, 154
Hand, 162–4
    see also Wrist and hand
Hip joint, 126–31
    joint play, 128–30
        external rotation, 130
        internal rotation, 130
        posterior shear, 130
    osseous landmark location, 127–9
    soft tissue landmark location, 127, 129
Humerus, 135, 146
    greater tubercle, 135, 138–9
    lesser tubercle, 135, 140

Iliotibial band, 118–19
Ilium, 126
Infraspinatus, 135
Inguinal ligament, 127, 129
Intermetatarsal joint, 110
Interpersonal issues, xvii
Intersegmental restriction, 15
Intervertebral joint fixation, 15
Ischial tuberosity, 127, 128
Ischium, 126

Joint challenge, 11
Joint play, 10, 11
    foot and ankle, 106–10
        intermetatarsals, 110
        metatarsophalangeal joint, 109–10
        subtalar joint, 109
        talocrural joint, 107–9
    hip joint, 128–30
        external rotation, 130
        internal rotation, 130
        posterior shear, 130
    knee, 121–5
        patellofemoral joint, 122–5
        tibiofemoral joint, 121–2
    shoulder girdle, 143–4
    wrist and hand, 158–67
        fingers, 162, 165–7
        metacarpals, 161–2
        palmar surface of hand, 162–4
        radiocarpal joint, 158, 159
        thumb, 162, 164
        wrist joint, 158–61
Joint play analysis
    lumbar spine
        counter-rotation specific, 61–3
        lateral to medial, 60–1
        posterior-anterior, 57–60
    static, 56–7

Kinematics, 12–14
    clinical considerations, 14
    degrees of freedom, 13–14
    right-handed cartesian coordinate system, 12–13

types of motion, 12–13
Kinetics, 12
Knee, 111–25
    active range of motion, 112–13
    joint play, 121–5
        patellofemoral joint, 122–5
        tibiofemoral joint, 121–2
    landmark location, 112–13
    osseous landmarks, 113–17
        adductor tubercle and medial epicondyle, 114
        head of fibula, 116, 117
        inferior surface of patella, 117, 118
        lateral femoral condyle, 116, 117
        lateral femoral epicondyle, 116, 117
        lateral tibial plateau, 115–16
        lateral tibial tubercle, 116
        medial femoral condyle, 113
        medial tibial plateau, 113
        patella, 114–15
        tibial condyle, 113
        tibial tubercle and patellar tendon, 113
        trochlear groove, 117, 118
    soft tissue landmarks
        ligamentous structures, 120–1
            lateral collateral ligament, 120, 121
            medial collateral ligament, 120–1
            medial and lateral meniscus, 121
        muscular structures, 118–20
            biceps femoris, 118, 119
            gracilis, 120
            iliotibial band, 118–19
            media and lateral head of gastrocnemius, 119–20
            pes anserine bursa, 120
            quadriceps, 118
            sartorius, 120
            semitendinosus, 120

Lateral collateral ligament, 102–3, 111, 120
Lateral epicondyle
    elbow, 148–52
    femoral, 116, 117
Lateral head, 135
Lateral meniscus, 111, 121
Lateral tibial plateau, 115, 116
Lateral tibial tubercle, 116
Lateral to medial joint play analysis, 60–1
Latissimus dorsi, 135
Legal issues, xvi–xvii
Lesser trochanter, 126
Levator scapula, 135
Long head, 135
Lower extremity palpation, 87–131
    foot and ankle, 89–110
    hip, 126–31
    knee, 111–25
Lumbar spine
    combined movement end play, 71–2
    extension end play, 71–2

joint play analysis
    counter-rotation specific, 61–3
    lateral to medial, 60–1
    posterior-anterior, 57–60
lateral bending end play, 68–71
rotation end play, 71
Lumbopelvic palpation, 45–72
    dynamic end play analysis, 63–72
        combined movement and play, 71–2
        pelvic complex and sacroiliac joint, 63–7
        thoracolumbar spine, 67–71
    lumbar spine
        counter-rotation specific joint play analysis, 61–3
        lateral to medial joint play analysis, 60–1
        posterior-anterior joint play analysis, 57–60
    soft tissue palpation and osseous landmark identification,
        48–56
    stance, 46–8
    static joint play analysis, 56–7
Lunate, 154

Malleolus
    lateral aspect, 98–9
    medial aspect, 94
Medial collateral ligament, 103, 111, 120–1
Medial epicondyle
    elbow, 147–8
    knee, 114, 115
Medial meniscus, 111, 121
Medial tibial plateau, 113
Metacarpal joint, 154, 161–2
Metatarsal joint, 89, 91–2, 96, 97
Metatarsophalangeal joint, 91, 96, 109–10
Motion palpation, xv
    definition, 3–4
    dynamic, 4–8
    reliability, 15–18
    validity, 18–19
Multangular bones, 154

Navicular (scaphoid), 154
Navicular tubercle, 89, 92, 93
Neutral zone, 13

Obturator foramen, 126
Olecranon, 147, 148
Os pubis, 126
Osseous landmarks
    cervicothoracic region, 81–5
    foot and ankle
        lateral aspect, 96–9
            cuboid, 96–7
            fifth metatarsal and styloid process, 96
            fifth metatarsophalangeal joint, 96
            lateral aspect of calcaneus, 97
            lateral malleolus, 98
        medial aspect, 91–5
            Achilles tendon, 94–5

Osseous landmarks (*continued*)
    Achilles tendon insertion, 94
    first (medial) cuneiform, 92
    first metatarsophalangeal joint, 91
    head of talus, 92, 93
    medial calcaneus, 94
    medial malleolus, 94
    metatarsals, 91–2
    navicular, 92
    sustentaculum tali, 94
  hip, 127–9
  knee, 113–17
    adductor tubercle and medial epicondyle, 114, 115
    head of fibula, 116, 117
    inferior surface of patella, 117, 118
    lateral femoral condyle, 116, 117
    lateral femoral epicondyle, 116, 117
    lateral tibial plateau, 115–16
    lateral tibial tubercle, 116
    medial femoral condyle, 113, 115
    medial tibial plateau, 113
    patella, 114–15, 116
    tibial condyle, 113
    tibial tubercle and patellar tendon, 113
    trochlear groove, 117, 118
  lumbopelvic palpation, 48–56
  scapular region, 77–8
  shoulder girdle, 136–41
    acromioclavicular joint, 136–8
    acromion, 138, 139
    bicipital groove, 139
    clavicle, 136, 137
    coracoid process, 140
    greater tubercle of humerus, 138–9
    lesser tubercle of humerus, 140
    sternoclavicular joint, 136

Passive accessory palpation, 8–11
Patella, 114–15, 116
  inferior surface, 117, 118
Patellar tendon, 113
Patellofemoral joint, 122–5
Pectoralis major, 141
Pelvic crest, 49–51
Peroneus brevis, 102
Peroneus longus, 102
Personal boundaries, violation of, xvi
Pes anserine bursa, 120
Phalanges, 89
Pisiform bone, 154
Popliteal artery, 106
Posterior cruciate ligament, 111
Posterior spinal palpation, 75–7
Posterior superior iliac spine, 19, 20, 49, 49–51
  static joint play analysis, 56–7
Posterior tibial artery, 106
Posterior-anterior joint play analysis, 57–60
Postural observation, 35–44

dynamic postural examination
  sitting, 41–3
    forward flexion, 41–2
    lateral flexion, 41–3
  standing, 39–41
    backward extension, lateral view, 41
    forward flexion, lateral view, 39–41
    lateral flexion, posterior-anterior view, 41
static postural examination, 36–9
  anterior-posterior view, 39–40
  lateral view, 39
  posterior-anterior view, 36–8
Posture for lumbopelvic palpation, 46–8
Proximal radio-ulnar joint, 146
PSIS *see* Posterior superior iliac spine

Quadriceps, 118

Radiocarpal joint, 158, 159
Radiohumeral joint, 146
Radius, 146, 154
Rhomboid major, 135
Rhomboid minor, 135
Rib spring, 62–3
Right-handed cartesian coordinate system, 12–13
Rotation, 12

Sacral inferior lateral angle, 19, 20
Sacral sulcus, 19, 20
Sacral tubercle, 49–51
Sacroiliac joints
  dynamic end play analysis, 63–7
    innominate (ischial) flare, 65–7
    lateral bending, 63–4
    nutation/counternutation, 65
    reciprocal innominate movement, 64–5
  static joint play analysis, 56–7
    PSIS contact, 56–7
    sacral contact, 57
Sartorius muscle, 120
Scapula, 135
  landmark palpation, 77–8
    inferior pole of scapula, 77–8
    spine of scapula, 77
Segmental identification, 19–22
Semitendinosus muscle, 120
Shoulder girdle, 135–45
  joint play, 143–4
  muscular landmarks, 140–3
    biceps brachii, 141–3
    deltoid, 142, 143
    pectoralis major, 141, 142
    sternocleidomastoid, 140, 141
    trapezius, 140, 141
  osseous landmarks, 136–40
    acromioclavicular joint, 136–8
    acromion, 138
    bicipital groove, 139

clavicle, 136, 137
coracoid process, 140
greater tubercle of humerus, 138–9
lesser tubercle of humerus, 140
sternoclavicular joint, 136
Soft tissue landmarks
hip, 127, 129
knee
ligamentous structures, 120–1
lateral collateral ligament, 120, 121
medial collateral ligament, 120–1
medial and lateral meniscus, 121
muscular structures, 118–20
biceps femoris, 118, 119
gracilis, 120
iliotibial band, 118, 119
medial and lateral head of gastrocnemius, 119–20
pes onserine bursa, 120
quadriceps, 118
sartorius, 120
semitendinosus, 120
plantar aspect of foot, 102–5
Achilles tendon, 103, 105
anterior talofibular ligament, 103
calcaneofibular ligament, 103
extensor digitorum longus, 102
extensor hallucis longus, 102
lateral collateral ligaments, 102–3
medial collateral ligament, 103
peroneus longus and brevis, 102
tibialis anterior, 102
Soft tissue palpation, 48–56
Specificity assumption, 19–22
Spinous process, 49–51
Splenius cervicis, 135
Static joint play analysis, 56–7
Static palpation, xv
definition, 2–6
Static postural examination, 36–9
anterior-posterior view, 39–40
lateral view, 39
posterior-anterior view, 36–8
Sternoclavicular joint, 136
Sternocleidomastoid muscle, 140, 141
Styloid process, 96, 97
Subtalar joint, 109
Superspinatus muscle, 135

Sustentaculum tali, 94, 95
Talocrural (tibiotalar) joint, 107–9
Talus, 89, 92, 93
Technique, xv
Teres major, 135
Teres minor, 135
Thoracic spine palpation, 73–8
anterior chest wall, 74–5
posterior spinal, 75–7
scapular region, 77–8
Thoracolumbar spine, dynamic end play analysis, 67–71
Thumb, 162, 164
Tibial condyle, 113
Tibial tubercle, 113
Tibialis anterior muscle, 102
Tibiofemoral joint, 121–2
Touch, issues surrounding, xvi
Translation, 12–13
Trapezius muscle, 140, 141
Triquetrium, 154
Trochlea, 146
Trochlear groove, 117

Ulna, 146, 152, 154
Ulno-humeral joint, 146
Upper extremity palpation, 133–4
elbow, 146–53
shoulder girdle, 135–45
wrist and hand, 154–67

Vascular structures
lower extremity, 105–6
dorsalis pedis artery, 105–6
popliteal artery, 106
posterior tibial artery, 106

Wrist and hand, 154–67
joint play, 158–67
fingers, 162, 165–7
metacarpals, 161–2
palmar surface of hand, 162–4
radiocarpal joint, 158, 159
thumb, 162, 164
wrist joint, 158–61
wrist region, 155–8
Wrist joint, 158–61